Female Genital Mutilation

Akintayo Odeyemi

Female Genital Mutilation

Reasons, Practice, Effects

VDM Verlag Dr. Müller

Imprint

Bibliographic information by the German National Library: The German National Library lists this publication at the German National Bibliography; detailed bibliographic information is available on the Internet at http://dnb.d-nb.de.
Any brand names and product names mentioned in this book are subject to trademark, brand or patent protection and are trademarks or registered trademarks of their respective holders. The use of brand names, product names, common names, trade names, product descriptions etc. even without a particular marking in this works is in no way to be construed to mean that such names may be regarded as unrestricted in respect of trademark and brand protection legislation and could thus be used by anyone.

Cover image: www.purestockx.com

Publisher:
VDM Verlag Dr. Müller Aktiengesellschaft & Co. KG , Dudweiler Landstr. 125 a, 66123 Saarbrücken, Germany,
Phone +49 681 9100-698, Fax +49 681 9100-988,
Email: info@vdm-verlag.de

Zugl.: Berrien Springs, Andrews University, Diss., 1996

Produced in USA and UK by:
Lightning Source Inc., La Vergne, Tennessee, USA
Lightning Source UK Ltd., Milton Keynes, UK
BookSurge LLC, 5341 Dorchester Road, Suite 16, North Charleston, SC 29418, USA

ISBN: 978-3-639-02464-7

TABLE OF CONTENTS

LIST OF ILLUSTRATIONS

LIST OF TABLES

LIST OF ABBREVIATIONS

AHI	Action Health Incorporated
CBO	Community Based Organization
CGSPS	Center for Gender and Social Policy Studies, Obafemi Awolowo University, Ile-Ife, Nigeria
CNN	Cable Network News
FGM	Female Genital Mutilation
HIV	Human Immunodeficiency Virus
HTP	Harmful Traditional Practice
IAC	Inter-African Committee
ICPD	International Conference on Population and Development
LGA	Local Government Area
MOH	Ministry of Health
NANNM	National Association of Nigerian Nurses and Midwives
NGO	Non-Governmental Organization
OAU	Organization of African Unity
TBA	Traditional Birth Attendant
UNDS	United Nations Development Systems
UNICEF	United Nations Children Funds
VRF	Vesico Rectum Fistula
VVF	Vesico Vagina Fistula
WIN	Women International Network
WHO	World Health Organization

ACKNOWLEDGMENTS

It is with some hesitation that I write these words of acknowledgment. This is due to the fear c the possibility of leaving out someone who played a significant role in the completion of this worl Many hands have come together to render direct and indirect assistance toward this achievement. thank God for each one of them.

This achievement would have been impossible without some people and organizations Gc directed my way. I thank God for my wife, Yetunde, who taught me to believe it could be done ar who brought in her own experience in the field to support. I am immensely grateful to ADR International, Rigmor Nyberg (ADRA Sweden's former Country Director), Dr. Greg Saunders, D Randy Skau, and ADRA Nigeria Board of Directors for the assistance rendered. My appreciation al goes to friends such as Dr. A. J. Farinde, late Dr. Ayo Awoyinka and Dimeji Babalola a form colleague in ADRA Nigeria.

I was blessed with a distinguished review committee in Andrews University. Jimmy Kijai, Li Beardsley, and Sten LaBianca became brothers and sister to me, spent their means and themselves seeing me through the research work. Without them, this book would have remained uncompleted. just cannot thank them enough.

FOREWORD

Preservation and continuation of cultural practices is needed for the identity of a people. However approaches for continuity of cultural practices should be weighed heavily against development and rights of people for which such practices have implications.

This research has critically looked into the reasons for the practice of Female Genital Mutilation or Cutting in spite of it being identified as having negative implications on reproductive rights as well as individual rights of the females on which it is performed. Using data collected from among a group in Nigeria with a reported high prevalence rate of FGM, the roles and identification of principal actors is examined along side possible of FGM practices on units of the society such as; the individual, household and marital units. Findings from this study indicate that the culture of secrecy on sexuality in the Africa culture is a great determinant for sustenance, continuity as well as support from those on which it is practiced. The necessity and compulsion of circumcising female children is stilled based on age long myths, such as the uncircumcised clitoris in contact with during child bearing results in instant death.

Due to it social and cultural acceptability both trained medical personnel and local practitioners are involved in the FGM operation for the gain of an extra income. Though women are the ones affected by FGM operations, this research shows that women are the ones who refuse to discuss its impacts and termination. Nearly half of the male respondents are in support of termination of the practice or modification of the procedure and type of FGM. Though FGM is a practice entrenched in culture, it is not immutable as adjustments and changes that will allow for developmental benefits can be achieved through education and sensitization programs.

This is indicative in this very research as the author; a man got exposed into the 'secrecy' of FGM. An exposure of its why, how, implications, and male opinion documented by a male researcher lays credence to the fact that its perpetuation is not just carried out to please men but for the desire upheld by society at large of both men and women.

Yetunde Odeyemi PhD
Technical Advisor, Programs and Planning,
ADRA Africa Regional Office,
Nairobi.

TABLE OF CONTENTS

i

LIST OF ILLUSTRATIONS

LIST OF TABLES

LIST OF ABBREVIATIONS

AHI	Action Health Incorporated
CBO	Community Based Organization
CGSPS	Center for Gender and Social Policy Studies, Obafemi Awolowo University, Ile-Ife, Nigeria
CNN	Cable Network News
FGM	Female Genital Mutilation
HIV	Human Immunodeficiency Virus
HTP	Harmful Traditional Practice
IAC	Inter-African Committee
ICPD	International Conference on Population and Development
LGA	Local Government Area
MOH	Ministry of Health
NANNM	National Association of Nigerian Nurses and Midwives
NGO	Non-Governmental Organization
OAU	Organization of African Unity
TBA	Traditional Birth Attendant
UNDS	United Nations Development Systems
UNICEF	United Nations Children Funds
VRF	Vesico Rectum Fistula
VVF	Vesico Vagina Fistula
WIN	Women International Network
WHO	World Health Organization

ACKNOWLEDGMENTS

It is with some hesitation that I write these words of acknowledgment. This is due to the fear of the possibility of leaving out someone who played a significant role in the completion of this work. Many hands have come together to render direct and indirect assistance toward this achievement. I thank God for each one of them.

This achievement would have been impossible without some people and organizations God directed my way. I thank God for my wife, Yetunde, who taught me to believe it could be done and who brought in her own experience in the field to support. I am immensely grateful to ADRA International, Rigmor Nyberg (ADRA Sweden's former Country Director), Dr. Greg Saunders, Dr. Randy Skau, and ADRA Nigeria Board of Directors for the assistance rendered. My appreciation also goes to friends such as Dr. A. J. Farinde, late Dr. Ayo Awoyinka and Dimeji Babalola a former colleague in ADRA Nigeria.

I was blessed with a distinguished review committee in Andrews University. Jimmy Kijai, Lisa Beardsley, and Sten LaBianca became brothers and sister to me, spent their means and themselves in seeing me through the research work. Without them, this book would have remained uncompleted. I just cannot thank them enough.

FOREWORD

Preservation and continuation of cultural practices is needed for the identity of a people. However approaches for continuity of cultural practices should be weighed heavily against development and rights of people for which such practices have implications.

This research has critically looked into the reasons for the practice of Female Genital Mutilation or Cutting in spite of it being identified as having negative implications on reproductive rights as well as individual rights of the females on which it is performed. Using data collected from among a group in Nigeria with a reported high prevalence rate of FGM, the roles and identification of principal actors is examined along side possible of FGM practices on units of the society such as; the individual, household and marital units. Findings from this study indicate that the culture of secrecy on sexuality in the Africa culture is a great determinant for sustenance, continuity as well as support from those on which it is practiced. The necessity and compulsion of circumcising female children is stilled based on age long myths, such as the uncircumcised clitoris in contact with during child bearing results in instant death.

Due to it social and cultural acceptability both trained medical personnel and local practitioners are involved in the FGM operation for the gain of an extra income. Though women are the ones affected by FGM operations, this research shows that women are the ones who refuse to discuss its impacts and termination. Nearly half of the male respondents are in support of termination of the practice or modification of the procedure and type of FGM. Though FGM is a practice entrenched in culture, it is not immutable as adjustments and changes that will allow for developmental benefits can be achieved through education and sensitization programs.

This is indicative in this very research as the author; a man got exposed into the 'secrecy' of FGM. An exposure of its why, how, implications, and male opinion documented by a male researcher lays credence to the fact that its perpetuation is not just carried out to please men but for the desire upheld by society at large of both men and women.

Yetunde Odeyemi PhD
Technical Advisor, Programs and Planning,
ADRA Africa Regional Office,
Nairobi.

1

CHAPTER ONE

INTRODUCTION

Background

The practice of Female Circumcision has cultural, maternal, and health consequences. According to Adebajo (1992), the majority, if not all, of the dangerous practices that are harmful to maternal health in all societies are performed under the auspices of traditional or cultural beliefs and inclinations. Traditional practices are norms of care and behavior based on age, lifestyle, gender and social class, which have been handed down through succeeding generation (United Nations Development Systems [UNDS], 1998). A good number of African traditional practices, such as moonlight dances and the use of chewing sticks, have their merits. Some have no known positive merits, but rather, are detrimental to the health and psychological and social well-being of people, especially of women and girls whose fundamental human rights are usually violated by these practices (UNDS, 1998). Due to the patriarchal nature of most societies in Africa, it is an established fact that most harmful practices are impacted mostly on either women or the female child (Center for Gender and Social Policy Studies [CGSPS], 1999). This is because, at the various levels of African society, women do not have a voice in decision-making; neither are they active policy makers. Rather, they are invisible. The extreme to be coped with in this situation, however, is the fact that although most traditional practices do not impact favorably on women, women are known to be strong and active agents and custodians of traditions. Thus, women play an active role in perpetuating and upholding tradition, and therefore, the harmful practices (CGSPS, 1999).

Harmful Traditional Practices (HTPs) were created and are being sustained by culture, custom, religion, mores, norms, and values of diverse ethnic groups (UNDS, 1998). The most common ones in Nigeria fall into three main categories: (1) reproductive health practices, (2) nutrition-related practices, and (3) human rights-associated practices.

The identified reproductive health practices include Female Circumcision, which is also referred to as Female Genital Mutilation (FGM). Others practices include: Yankari, Gishiri or salt cut; hot bath; early marriage and pregnancy; total privacy during labor; the use of herbs and charms to control fertility; fatalistic and supernaturalistic attitudes to childbirth; and forced squatting during labor.

Nutrition-related practices are abstinence from some proteinous foods during pregnancy, childbirth, and during breast feeding, and food taboos that disallow children from being served nutritious food because it is believed that it might encourage the habit of stealing. An example of practices related to human-rights is that females are not allowed to take decisions on reproductive health, male child preference, inheritance practices, and widowhood rites (UNDS, 1998).

The World Health Organization (WHO; 1997) defines female circumcision as comprising "all procedures involving partial or total removal of the external female genitalia or other injury to the female genital organs whether for cultural or other non-therapeutic reasons" (p. 3). If mutilation is seen as a definitive and irremediable removal of any healthy organ, then based on WHO's definition of female circumcision, the term Female Genital Mutilation (FGM) is an appropriate one.

FGM constitutes violence against the rights of women and children in the sense that the victim has no say over it. It is usually performed early in life. What complicates the issue is that it is mothers who assist their children or grandchildren to undergo the operation.

2

The act has not abated in spite of studies and a few pockets of interventions. To eradicate it, there is a need to know the opinion of those involved and give them say in arriving at possible solutions. The eradication of FGM involves a change. And change as a development principle must be participatory to be sustainable.

The results of a national baseline survey of positive and harmful traditional practices against women, commissioned by the Federal Government of Nigeria and the United Nations Development Systems (UNDS, 1998), and conducted by the Center for Gender and Social Policy Studies, Obafemi Awolowo University, Ile-Ife, Nigeria, showed that FGM is practiced by 32.9% of households in Nigeria. However, the highest rates were found to be in the States of Osun (98.7%), Oyo (96.8%), and Ondo (91.6%) (UNDS, 1998). All these states are in the Yoruba territory in the southwest of Nigeria.

In many cultures in Africa, sexuality as a topic is an obscure area, which is hardly discussed except for very specific reasons. This has been one of the reasons why Female Genital Mutilation remains undiscussed in many circles. The silence over it in turn assists in perpetuating the practice. Many writers have tied the practice of FGM to the position of women in society (Adebajo, 1992; Koso-Thomas, 1987; Owumi, 1994). Until very recently when pockets of intervention efforts started, the practice of FGM was not presented to women in a straightforward manner. In most of the society, it is shrouded in mystery, magic, and fear. As it is among the Efiks in southeastern Nigeria (UNDS, 1998), women receive social approval when they undergo the practice and gain certain benefits such as being marriageable and thus having access to resources in the community. Because of the social disapproval and the sanctions women face if they do not undergo FGM, they inevitably end up viewing it in a positive light. This is because the practice is strongly linked to virginity, chastity, and fidelity, which are prerequisites for marriage.

Koso-Thomas (1987) observed that the right to belong, to be accepted in a community ought not to be purchased at such a high price in human suffering. Thus, the problem needs to be well understood by understanding the knowledge, beliefs, and practice of those who are affected by it, and the various actors involved with FGM.

Although no specific and direct study on FGM had been carried out in the study area, the national research commissioned by the UNDS and carried out by the Center for Gender and Social Policy Studies of Obafemi Awolowo University in 1996/1997 has some influence over the people.

Purpose of the Study

The purpose of this research was to look into the practice of FGM among a group of people with a high prevalence rate in Ife East Local Government Area (LGA) of Osun State in Nigeria. The study will:
1. Identify the possible origin of female genital circumcision
2. Identify the reasons for the practice and the prevailing type(s) of practice
3. Identify the principal actors and their roles in FGM
4. Examine the possible effects on households and marriage.

These activities were carried out among the inhabitants of the Ife East Local Government Area of Osun State in Nigeria.

The study was guided by the following research questions:
1. What are the beliefs of the respondents about Female Genital Mutilation?

2. What is the level of the respondents' knowledge about FGM?
3. What are the reasons for practicing FGM?
4. What is the prevalence rate of FGM in the study area?
5. Which types of FGM are practiced in the study area?
6. At what age is FGM usually carried out in the study area?
7. Who are the FGM practitioners in the study area?
8. How are the practitioners paid for the operations performed?
9. What instruments are used in the operation?
10. What post-operation care is given?
11. What are the post-operation complications?
12. What is the attitude of men about marriage to uncircumcised females?
13. What are the effects of FGM on men?
14. What is the attitude of the people toward modification and eradication of FGM?

This study contributes to having firsthand information on the knowledge, beliefs, and practice of a group of people whose prevalence rate of FGM is asserted to be over 98% (UNDS, 1998). Knowledge of the types practiced, why it is practiced, the hazards involved, and the people's contribution provides a basis for developing an eradication plan.

Thus, an intervention program in the community might be developed and this replicated in other communities within Osun State and other areas with high rates of FGM practices.

This study also constitutes a male voice contribution to the practice of FGM. It has been said that it is perpetuated because men still want it.

The cultural setting of the Yorubas makes this type of study quite difficult because the topic is hardly discussed at home or even among peers. Some questions could only be asked indirectly and only by female interviewers. Thus, focus group discussions, which were participatory, were used to elicit information that would not be divulged openly in heterogeneous groups.

4

CHAPTER TWO

LITERATURE REVIEW

General Historical Background

Throughout human history, mankind has developed many customs and traditions that are related to social organization and cultural codes of behavior (Abdalla, 1982). Oke (1997) defined culture as "social heredity or the things men (and children and women) learn when they are trained within a particular group of people" (p. 15), and defined tradition as cultural continuity transmitted in the form of social attitudes, beliefs, principles and conventions of behavior deriving from past experience and viewed as a convention established by constant practices. A belief or legend based on oral report usually accepted as historically true, though without evidence. (Oke, 1997, p. 15)

Female Genital Mutilation, sometimes referred to as Female Circumcision, is one of the deeply rooted traditional practices with severe health implications for girls and women (WHO, 1997).

There has been a lot of misinformation regarding the terminology Female Circumcision and what the practice entails. Therefore it took some time for writers to adopt the term Female Genital Mutilation in contrast to the euphemistic term Female Circumcision (Dorkenoo, 1994). However, the United Nations General Assembly overwhelmingly rejected the term Female Circumcision' in describing FGM because of the gross disparities between removal of the male foreskin and that of the female genitalia (Negerie, 1997). This is because any definitive and irremediable removal of a healthy organ constitutes a mutilation.

FGM is a complex social practice which is defined by WHO (1997) as comprising "all procedures involving partial or total removal of the external female genitalia or other injury to the female genital organs whether for cultural or other non-therapeutic reasons." (p. 3). Different types of FGM have been identified in various countries. Each of the various types has not only been given different descriptions, but even different names in some cases. This made it necessary that there be standardization of the different types and descriptions in literature as put in place by the WHO.

The origins of FGM are unknown (Badri, 1972; WHO, 1996). Negerie (1997) described FGM as a procedure that has been in existence for about 5,000 years, dating back to ancient Egypt. In the past, it was practiced by many cultures, including those of the Phoenicians, Hittites, and the ancient Egyptians (Koso-Thomas, 1987).

Female Genital Mutilation is known to have been practiced in virtually all continents of the world (Oke, 1997). It is, however, more connected with African countries, and migrants from this continent are believed to have introduced it in the other continents as continental migration grew in scope (Adebajo, 1992). In 1769, Niebuhr, a German traveler, reported that in Oman, the shores of the Persian Gulf, among the Christians of Abyssinia, in Egypt, and among the Arabs and Copts, this custom was prevalent (Baasher, 1979). Herodotus alluded to Female Genital Mutilation as early as 500 B.C. (Rushwan, 1990).

Many people think that FGM has Islamic roots (CGSPS, 1999). However, the practice was well known and widespread in some areas of the world including the Arab Peninsula before the Islamic era. This means that female circumcision could not have been an Islamic custom. Negerie (1997) also disagreed with the possibility of FGM being founded on Islamic injunction. To Negerie (1997) a Pharaonic rather than Islamic origin is more likely to be acceptable. This point is strengthened by the fact that Type III of FGM, which is referred to as infibulation, is also otherwise known as "Pharaonic circumcision."

Various kinds of acts amounting to FGM have been performed in many cultures to repress female sexuality. Koso-Thomas (1987) reported that early Romans used a technique of slipping rings through the labia majora of female slaves as a barrier against pregnancy, while a chastity belt was introduced in Europe in the 12th century by the Crusaders to prevent unlawful or unsanctioned sex. Modern physicians in England and the United States as recently as the 1940s and 1950s used FGM to treat hysteria, lesbianism, masturbation, and some other female deviancies (Koso-Thomas, 1987)

Prevalence and Distribution

In 1996, WHO reported a lack of availability of comprehensive country-by-country data of FGM. The only nationwide survey data available at that time were from the Sudan, Cote d'Ivoire, and Central African Republic. However, in 1998 the report of a study on harmful and positive traditional practices that affect women and girls in Nigeria, funded by the United Nations Development System (UNDS, 1998) and carried out by the Center for Gender and Social Policy Studies, Ile-Ife, Nigeria, was released. The report gave comprehensive statistics on the prevalence of FGM and other Harmful Traditional Practices (HTP) in Nigeria according to the different States in the country.

WHO's (1996) estimate claimed that, around the world, there were between 100 and 132 million girls and women who have been subjected to FGM. (See Fig. 1.) Each year, a further 2 million girls are estimated to be at risk of the practice. A vast majority of such girls live in 28 African countries, as shown in Table 1, a few in the Middle East and Asian countries, and increasingly in Europe, Canada, Australia, New Zealand and the United States.

In South America, FGM is practiced in Brazil, Eastern Mexico and Peru (Koso-Thomas, 1987). Koso-Thomas also speculated that the ethnic groups who settled in Brazil following the abolition of the slave trade in the 19th century might have imported the practice there from West Africa. This is an acceptable probability as West African settlers in the central part of Brazil retained many of their former cultural practices. One such cultural practice that is still found among the Yorubas of southwest Nigeria is the similarities in the modes of worship of *Olokun,* the water goddess (and the deity also regarded as the goddess of fertility), and *Ogun,* the god of iron. This thought is strengthened by the fact that the people in the central part of Brazil speak the Yoruba language (Koso-Thomas, 1987). While FGM is practiced in Muslim regions of the United Arab Emirate, South Yemen, Bahrain, and Oman, it is not found in Saudi Arabia, the seat of Islam (Negerie, 1997).

6

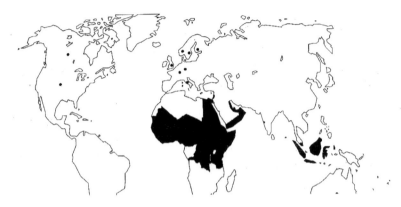

Fig. 1: Areas of the world in which FGM has been reported to occur.

From "Female Genital Mutilation: A joint WHO/UNICEF/UNFPA Statement." By World

Health Organization, 1997, Geneva: World Health Organization, p.6.

TABLE 1:

ESTIMATED PREVALENCE OF FEMALE GENITAL
MUTILATION IN AFRICA

	Country	Estimated Prevalence	No. of Women ('000) **	Source of Prevalence Rate
1	Benin*	50%	1,370	
2	Burkina Faso	70%	3,650	Report of the National Committee (1995).
3	Cameroon	20%	1,330	Estimated prevalence based on a study (1994) in southwest and far north provinces by the Inter-African Committee, Cameroon section.
4	Central African Republic	43%	740	National Demographic and Health Survey (1994/1995). Signs of decline among younger age groups. Secondary or higher education can be associated with reduced rates of FGM. No significant variations between rural and urban rates. The prevalence of FGM is highest amongst the Banda and Mandjia groups where 84% and 71% of women respectively have undergone FGM.
5	Chad	60%	1,930	1990 and 1991 UNICEF sponsored studies in three regions.
6	Cote d'Ivoire	43%	3,020	National Demographic and Health Survey (1994). A reduced rate of FGM among younger women. No significant variations occurred between urban and rural rates. Secondary and higher education can be associated with reduced rates of FGM. The highest prevalence of FGM appears amongst the Muslim population (80%), compared with 15% among Protestants and 17% among Catholics.
7	Djibouti*	98%	290	Type III widely practiced, UN ECOSOC Report (1991).
8	Egypt*	80%	24,710	Type I and Type II practiced by both Muslims

8

and Christians. Types III, infibulation reported
in areas of south Egypt closer to Sudan.

Table 1 – *Continued.*

9	Eritrea*	90%	1,600	
10	Ethiopia	85%	23,240	A 1995 UNICEF sponsored survey in five regions and an Inter-African Committee survey in twenty administrative regions. Type I and Type II commonly practiced by Muslims and Coptic Christians as well as by the Ethiopian Jewish population, most of who now live in Israel. Type III is common in areas bordering Sudan and Somalia.
11	Gambia	80%	450	A limited study by the Women's Bureau (1985). Type II common.
12	Ghana	30%	2,640	Pilot studies in the Upper East region (1996), and among migrant settlement in Accra (1987), by the Accra Association of Women's Welfare.
13	Guinea*	50%	1,670	
14	Guinea-Bissau	50%	270	Limited 1990 survey by the Union democratique des Femmes de la Guinee-Bisau.
15	Kenya	50%	7,050	A 1992 Maendeleo Ya Wanawake survey in four regions. Types I and II commonly practiced. Type III by a few groups. Decreasing in urban, but remains strong in rural Areas
16	Liberia*	60%	900	
17	Mali*	75%	4,110	
18	Mauritania*	25%	290	
19	Niger*	20%	930	
20	Nigeria	50%	28,170	A study by the Nigerian Association of Nurses and Nurse-midwives conducted in 1985-1986 showed that 13 out of the then 21 States had populations practicing FGM, prevalence ranging 35% to 90%. Types I and II

9

Table 1 – *Continued.*

commonly practiced.

21	Senegal	20%	830	Report of a national study by ENDA (1991).
22	Sierra Leone	90%	2,070	All ethnic groups practice FGM except for Christian Krios in the western region and in the capital, Freetown. Type II commonly practiced.
23	Somalia	98%	4,580	FGM is generally practiced; approximately 80% of the operations are infibulation.
24	Sudan	89%	12,450	National Demographic and Health Survey (1989/1990). A very high prevalence, predominantly infibulation, throughout most of the northern, northeastern, and northwestern regions. Along with a small overall decline in the 1980s, there is a shift from infibulation to clitoridectomy.
25	Togo*	50%	1,050	
26	Uganda*	5%	540	
27	United Republic of Tanzania*	10%	1,500	
28	Zaire*	5%	1,110	
	Total		**132,490**	

* Anecdotal information only; no published studies.
** Number of women calculated (in thousands) by applying the prevalence rate to the 1995 total female population reported in the United Nations Population Division population projections (1994 revision). Total may not add up due to rounding.
From *Female Genital Mutilation: Prevalence and Distribution*, by World Health Organization, August 1996, Geneva: World Health Organization.

The Practice

There are different types of FGM. To enhance an understanding of the different types, some elementary knowledge of the anatomy and physiology of the female genitalia is necessary. As shown in Fig. 2, the female genitalia consist of mons Veneris, labial majora, labia minora, clitoris, urethral opening, vagina, hymen, and the perineum (Koso-Thomas, 1987).

The *mons Veneris* is a mass of fatty tissues covering the pubic bone and is usually covered with hair, which forms a transverse hairline across the abdomen. The *labia majora* are outer skin (or big lips) of the genitalia; this and the inner skin fold, labia minora (or the small lip), cover and protect the opening of the vagina and urinary opening. The labia majora contain hair follicles, sebaceous glands, and subcutaneous fat. The *labia minora* have no hair follicles and consist of connective tissues containing little fat, and richly supplied with nerves, blood vessels and sebaceous glands. The upper end forms a hood of skin called the prepuce. The inner surfaces of the labiae majora and minora are kept moist by glandular secretions, which lubricate the inside of the skin folds and prevent soreness when they rub against each other.

The *clitoris* is a bud-shaped organ located under the hood formed by the labia minora. It is a very sensitive, erectile organ with a rich supply of nerve fibers and blood vessels. Because of these the clitoris swells and becomes erect when excited, and it is this excitement which causes female orgasm.

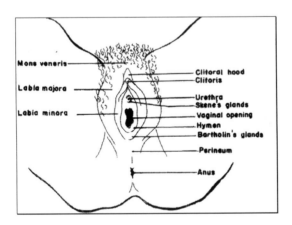

Fig. 2: Normal vulva before circumcision.

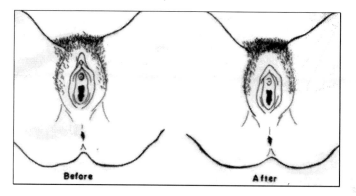

Before **After**

Fig. 3: Type I (*Sunna*)

The WHO (1996) has recognized four different types of FGM:

Type 1: *Clitoridectomy* is the excision of the prepuce of the clitoris with or without excision of part or the entire clitoris. This type is also referred to as "sunna."

Type 2: *Excision* (Fig. 3) is the removal of the prepuce, the clitoris itself and all or part of the labia minora, leaving the labia majora intact, and the rest of the vulva un-sutured. Both Types I and II constitute up to 80% of all procedures

Type 3: *Infibulation*. (Fig. 5) is the removal of the prepuce, the whole of labiae minora and majora, and the stitching together of the two sides of the vulva, leaving a very small orifice to permit the flow of urine and menstrual discharge.

Type 4: *Unclassified*. This includes pricking, piercing, or incision of clitoris and/or labia; stretching of clitoris and/or labia; cauterization by burning of clitoris and surrounding tissues; scraping (angurya cuts) of the vaginal orifice or cutting (Gishiri cuts) of the vagina; introduction of corrosive substances into the vagina to cause bleeding, or herbs into the vagina with the aim of tightening or narrowing the vagina (Action Health Incorporated, 1997).

According to the WHO report, Types I and II are the most common procedures. They constitute up to 80% of all the procedures. Type III, infibulation, is the most extreme form, and it constitutes approximately 15% of all procedures. Infibulation involves the complete removal of the clitoris and the labia minora as well as the inner surface of the labia majora. The two sides of the vulva are then stitched together with thorns, silk, or catgut sutures so that when the remaining skin of the labia majora heals, it forms a bridge of scar tissue over the vagina. A small opening is preserved by the insertion of a foreign body to allow for the passage of urine and menstrual blood.   The girl's legs are sometimes bound together from thigh to ankle and she may be immobilized from between 7 days, in some communities (Hosken, 1979), to several weeks to allow scar tissue to form over the wound. When the wound has healed, the reconstructed opening is surrounded by skin and tough scar tissue. If the vulva does not heal successfully or the opening is too big, the girl is operated on again.

12

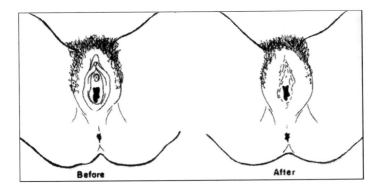

Fig. 4. Type II (*Excision*)

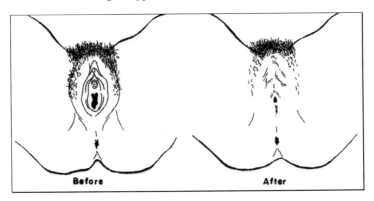

Fig. 5: Type III Infibulation (Pharaonic circumcision)

Since a physical barrier to intercourse has been created, the infibulated woman has to undergo gradual dilation by the husband after marriage. This is very painful and may take several days. Sometimes it is not possible for the husband to penetrate at all, and the opening has to be re-cut. At childbirth, the trauma of mutilation is repeated. The woman has to be defibulated to allow the passage of the baby. The passage can cause obstructed labor due to tough scar tissue surrounding the birth canal. After birth, the raw edges are sutured in the same way again. This is referred to as re-infibulation. According to Okunade (1997), re-infibulation is done for women who earlier experienced the Pharaonic circumcision after each childbirth, divorce, and on the death of their husband.

The operation of female circumcision is usually performed between the 8th day and 9 years. In Sudan, Nigeria, and many other developing countries, 74% of the girls were circumcised before the age of 9 years and 84% before their 10th birthday (UNDS, 1998). In Sudan, almost 81% of the girls had the operation done prior to their 8th birthday (Badri, 1983; Rushwan, 1990) and before the girl begins menstruation (Hetata, 1997). The age of circumcision differs widely in many areas of Nigeria. In the southwestern part of Nigeria, female circumcision is usually carried out within the first 8 days of birth (UNDS, 1998). In the Niger Delta region of Nigeria, it is performed on girls between 12 and 18 years old during an annual festival referred to as *Essim Ngbopo* (UNDS, 1998). According to the report of a national survey carried out by the National Association of Nigerian Nurses and Midwives (NANNM) between December 1985 and May 1986, the operation is performed in the 7th month of pregnancy in Bendel State (now reorganized into Edo and Delta States). In some of the States in the southeastern part of the country, it is performed on adolescent girls and adult women as part of puberty and initiation rites into womanhood. Such rites cover a period of 3 to 6 weeks during which the young women are taught housewifery, care of babies, and proper behavior towards in-laws (Adebajo, 1992).

Female Genital Mutilation is performed by different practitioners in the different areas where the practice is common. Traditionally, in many communities, the role of the practitioner is an inherited one (Jacobs, 1993), including skilled or unskilled, women or men usually between the ages of 35 and 70 years (Adebajo, 1992). In Sierra Leone, practitioners are highly respected female opinion leaders who have great influence over the traditional secret societies (Koso-Thomas, 1987). These people are considered to be priestesses (Jacobs, 1993). In northern Nigeria, it is done by the local barbers who usually are responsible for all traditional surgery, including all forms of tribal marks and incisions. Among the Yorubas, the *Olola* families are the traditional practitioners, and the trade is handed over from one generation to another (Action Health Incorporated [AHI], 1997). Owumi (1994) noted that an attempt to modernize FGM and respond to those who criticize the practice has led to its being taken over by modern health care providers. This is despite the fact that medical opinion is against FGM (CGSPS, 1999).

According to Jacobs (1993), the vested interests of many practitioners play a vital role in the continuation and spread of the practice. For example, in Sudan, Gambia, and Nigeria, practitioners include trained health personnel; however, most practitioners are from poverty-ridden backgrounds or families and/or ethnic groups, and with low social status, while some do it as a means of a second pay packet (Jacobs, 1993; UNDS, 1998). The income from FGM especially for the practitioner who dwells in the rural area is usually more than what other activities would bring. Therefore the increase in income from a valued service results in improved social status (UNDS, 1998). Therefore, it will require a lot of effort to persuade the practitioners to abandon the practice on the basis of humanitarian appeals without

14

adequate compensation (Owumi, 1994).

Instruments used in operation range from special knives, for example, a saw-toothed knife in Mali (Dorkenoo, 1994), to razor blades, for example, Moos el Shurfa in Sudan (Dorkenoo, 1994), or even sharp stones, also in Sudan (Dareer, 1982). Others include scissors, scalpels, glass, and razor blades (WHO, 1996). According to the WHO report, the use of anesthetic and antiseptics is uncommon. After the 15-to-20 minute's procedure, "paste mixtures made of herbs, local porridge, ashes, or other mixtures" are applied to the wound to stop bleeding.

Reasons for the Practice

The reasons adduced for the practices of FGM are varied and many. In many places, it is done because of the belief that a baby is bound to die during childbirth if its head touches the clitoris (Adebajo, 1992). Adebajo also reported that uncircumcised women are feared to harbor evil spirits from which they are freed only through circumcision. Other reasons for the practice include preservation of virginity and desirability for marriage, cure for infertility, and it may be carried out as a religious injunction (AHI, 1997). Despite the obvious negative effects of FGM and the campaign against its practice, four reasons have been advanced for its persistence in many societies (Badri, 1979). These are:

1. Ignorance of the public, especially mothers and grandmothers, as to the immediate and later danger of female circumcision
2. Lack/insufficiency of health education and basic health services
3. A widespread but false belief that FGM is endorsed by religion
4. Some issues based on a set of social values. These include:
   a. Virginity at marriage for women as a requirement in Sudanese and some other societies
   b. The belief that female circumcision prevents promiscuity and ensures virginity at marriage
   c. The belief that men prefer women to be circumcised and, hence, uncircumcised women will not be married
   d. The attitude of men that female circumcision is a women's concern or a mother's decision and, therefore, men assume a passive role in decisions concerning circumcision of their daughters
   e. The common language called cleansing or purifying operation.

Effects of the Practice of FGM

The complications and consequences of the practice of FGM on the victims are both immediate and life-long (Kiragu, 1995; WHO, 1997). However, whether immediate or long-term, the health consequences vary according to the type and severity of the procedure (WHO, 1997), and on the proficiency of the practitioner, the bluntness of the instrument used, and the struggles of the victim (Kiragu, 1995).

The immediate health consequences begin with excruciating pain because the procedure is often carried out without any anesthesia (Kiragu, 1995). The pain, as well as the hemorrhage from the operation usually, results in shock for the victim (Kiragu, 1995; Okunade, 1997; Owumi, 1997, WHO, 1997). Other recorded immediate consequences of the procedure include infections and urine retention (Kiragu, 1995; Okunade, 1997). Any of the complications may be fatal (WHO, 1997; Women International Network [WIN], 1993). Of recent there had been some anxiety over the possibility of HIV transmission where the same instrument is used over and over again without being treated, (Kiragu, 1995; WIN, 1993) and where infibulation encourages anal intercourse as an alternative to vaginal intercourse (WHO, 1997).

Long-term consequences of FGM include formation of tough scar tissue, keloids, and cysts (Kiragu, 1995), damage to urethra resulting in urinary incontinence, painful sexual experience, sexual dysfunction (Okunade, 1997; WHO, 1997), and infertility arising from pelvic inflammatory diseases caused by infection of the vagina, urinary tract, and pelvis (WHO, 1986). The WHO (1986) report observed that about 25% of infertility in Sudan was attributed to Pharaonic circumcision.

There are also some psychosexual and psychological health consequences. WHO (1997) and Okunade (1997) reported that FGM in whatever form results in sexual dysfunction in both partners following painful intercourse and reduced sexual sensitivity caused by clitoridectomy and narrowing of the virginal opening. The WHO (1997) report stated further:

Genital mutilation may leave a lasting mark on the life and mind of the woman who has undergone it. The psychological complications may be submerged deep in the child's subconscious and may trigger behavioral disturbances. The loss of trust and confidence in caregivers has been reported as a possible serious effect. In the long term, women may suffer feelings of incompleteness, anxiety, depression, chronic irritability and frigidity. They may experience marital conflicts. Many girls and women, traumatized by their experience but with no acceptable means of expressing their fears, suffer in silence. (p. 8)

FGM and Food Security

The value put on the practice of FGM in many societies where it is practiced is so high that even young girls usually volunteered for it, if given a choice. This is because they consider it a thing of pride to be circumcised (Owumi, 1993, 1994). Hendsbee (1998) declared that such a behavior is by virtue of a lack education and resources needed to see them through life. The African girl or woman did not reach this position because she is lazy (UNDS, 1998). She works from sun up to sun down, not only at home, but also on the farm. She is the first to wake, and the last to sleep (CGSPS, 1999). Unfortunately, all these efforts are unrecognized, making the typical African woman invisible, when community development is considered. She is invisible and vulnerable because she is landless (CGSPS, 1998). Thus, she depends on her parents, and when married, her husband, for life's necessities (Hendsbee, 1998). This puts a lot of importance on girls' ability to get married. Unfortunately, if a girl is not circumcised in many cultures where it is practiced, marriage will be impossible, and such a girl becomes an outcast in the society (Althaus, 1997; Dorkenoo, 1992). Thus, since FGM is considered an essential part of a woman's identity in many cultures, going contrary has serious social implications, which affect food security.

FGM usually have serious health consequences (Koso-Thomas, 1987; WHO 1996, 1997). The short and long-term consequences may directly result in depression and anxiety (WHO, 1997). "Their chronic health problems, infertility or loss of husband's attention due to difficult penetration, usually causes the depression." (Hendsbee, 1998, p. 2). Unfortunately, in many societies where the practice is common, polygamy is allowed. Ebomoyi (1987) reported that in Shao and Okelele communities of Kwara State in Nigeria, while a female can have only one husband, the male is free to be polygamous. This is true for the entire Yoruba land. On the other hand, contrary to popular belief, a woman has no guarantee of secure marriage even after undergoing mutilation. This is because at the end of

16

the day, the husband will likely be unsatisfied with her sexually (Hendsbee, 1998), or she develops infertility problems (WHO, 1997) which infibulated women are prone to. Both are grounds for divorce in Africa (Abusharaf, 1998). With a loss of health and husband, such a woman may never be food secured.

According to the World Bank (1994), good health is basic to human welfare and a fundamental objective of social and economic development. The World Bank (1994) also sees the effects of poor health as going far beyond physical pain and suffering. This is because poor health disturbs learning and production (World Bank, 1994). WHO (1997) believes that the issue of FGM must be addressed, if economic development needs of girls and women in FGM societies are to be met.

FGM and Human Rights

According to the Population Reference Bureau (1996), the 1994 International Conference on Population and Development (ICPD) recognized Female Genital Mutilation as a dangerous and medically unwarranted practice that violates the rights of girls. In a book jointly published by UNICEF and Nigeria's Federal Ministry of Women Affairs and Social Development, it was stated that the United Nation Convention on the Rights of the Child was adopted by the General Assembly on the 20th of November 1989. The aim was to improve the quality of life of children worldwide, enhance their dignity, protect their inalienable rights, and ultimately mobilize and focus global attention on their physical, mental, moral, and spiritual development (UNICEF/FMWASD, 1995).

Some of the basic principles of Children's Rights speak directly and indirectly against the practice of FGM. A few of such Articles include:

Article Five: "Every Child is entitled to protection from any act that interferes with his or her privacy, honor and reputation."

Article Nine: "Every Child must be protected from indecent and inhuman treatment through sexual exploitation, drug abuse, child labor, torture, maltreatment and neglect."

Article Four (Right to Communicate): "Every child has right to freely express ideas, opinions and thought on any issue concerning his or her interest, subject to restriction under the law." This article may be interpreted to mean that children should be allowed an informed say on the FGM. And to do this, infants should not be mutilated.

Under Section 17 (1) (b) of the 1979 Nigerian Constitution, it is provided that the sanctity of the human person shall be recognized and human dignity shall be maintained and enhanced. Pursuant to this, Section 31 of the Constitution also guarantees the right to dignity of the human person. Thus, no person shall be subjected to torture or to inhuman or degrading treatment. Unfortunately, the expression "inhuman or degrading treatment" is not defined by the Constitution. It is therefore left to the court to define what would amount to such a treatment (Akinyele-George, 1997).

Efforts toward the Elimination of FGM

While commenting on the Nigerian Constitution and FGM, Akinyele-George (1997) concluded that the issue of FGM is more sociological than legal. Kiragu (1995) believed that laws alone will not end FGM, though such laws illustrate government commitment to the eradication of FGM. In view of this, many attempts have been made to put an end to the

17

practice.

Legislative Actions

Many efforts have been made to eliminate FGM through legislation. In Ghana, the Criminal Code of 1960 (Act 29 A) states that whoever excises, infibulates, or otherwise mutilates female genital organs in whole or in part shall be guilty of a second-degree felony, and liable on conviction to imprisonment of not less than 3 years. (WIN, 1999). Kiragu (1995) reported that the National Government's campaign to eliminate FGM in Burkina Faso began in 1988. And for the entire continent of Africa, in September 1997, the Organization of African Unity (OAU) decided that "by the year 2000, concrete mechanisms for the implementation of a national policy shall be established and legislation for the elimination of all forms of violence against women and girl children especially female genital mutilation will have been enacted." (WIN,1998, p. 1). The *WIN News* also reported OAU as directing that "all countries shall immediately review existing policies and legislation and report to IAC the status of such policies and legislation relating to women and girl children particularly female genital mutilation, early marriage and widowhood rites (WIN, 1998a, p. 1).

However, the level of success with the legislation is suspect. Despite all the efforts made in Ghana, the *Ghanaian Times* (cited in WIN 1998b) reported that "a participant in a recent seminar on female genital mutilation suggested that doctors be made to perform the inhuman practice" to make it safe (WIN 1999, p. 1). *WIN News* (1994) also reported that when asked to comment on a CNN presentation on female genital mutilation, the Egyptian President claimed to have thought that the practice had disappeared in his country, while an Egyptian weekly, *Al Wafd*, claimed that several thousand girls were mutilated daily in Egypt. In a separate CNN interview, after being confronted with the facts and asked why the practice had not been prohibited, President Mubarak answered: "But we cannot pass such legislation as no one would follow it" (WIN, 1994, p. 1).

Educational Efforts

According to Okunade (1997), an aggressive pursuit of female education would raise awareness of women and also broaden their view to the need to resist continuous violation of their bodies and dignity. He concluded that legislation against the practice might likely drive it underground and thereby compound the problem. Kiragu (1995) also believed that mere legislation might be counterproductive. This conclusion has been proved by the Egyptian experience. Chelala (1998) reported that despite government's efforts, many women in Egypt still support FGM. Chelala therefore suggested that prohibition be accompanied by sustained educational efforts at grassroots and community levels.

Kiragu (1995) reported that education has been an important component of the efforts to eradicate FGM. He reported educational efforts in Burkina Faso, Kenya, Mali, Tanzania (WIN, 1993), Sudan, Somali (Sarau, 1998), and Nigeria. *WIN News* (1998a) also recorded a successful effort among the Sabim people of Uganda. In Nigeria, the National Association of Nigerian Nurses and Midwives (NANNM) has been educating the public through plays and other life performances (Kiragu, 1995).

The *Women International Network (WIN) News* is included in one of the most current efforts toward the eradication of FGM all over the world. According to the *WIN News* (autumn 1997), educational materials are being offered to all international and local organizations/groups sponsoring programs in African countries.

18

Alternatives to FGM

The practitioners' role is important in the eradication of FGM (Koso-Thomas, 1987; Owumi, 1993). In recognition of this, Kiragu (1995) reported that projects are being implemented to provide alternative jobs for the practitioners. One of these in Ghana has been training practitioners to become Traditional Birth Attendants (TBAs), while another in Ethiopia trained them in sandal making and bread baking (Kiragu, 1995). Chelala (1998) also reported the creation of an alternative rite in Kenya. The rite is called *Ntanira Na Mugambo* or "Circumcision through words." The rite involves a weeklong program, which includes counseling, training, and provision of information to young women. The program ends with the "coming of age" day, when the community members gather to have a celebration. According to Chalala, since August 1996 when it was started, about 300 women have passed through the experience as an alternative to the traditional mutilation.

CHAPTER THREE

METHODOLOGY

The Study Area

The study was carried out in Ife East Local Government Area (LGA) of Osun State, in southwest Nigeria. Ife East Local Government Area is one of the four LGAs in Ife land and it is also one of the 30 LGAs in Osun State. It had a population of 116,856 people (Osun State MOH). It covers an area of about 162.75 square kilometers. The southwestern part of Nigeria is traditionally inhabited the Yoruba people. See Fig. 6 and Fig. 7.

Ile-Ife history is wrapped up in many legends or myths that ascribe to it some unique characteristics among Yoruba towns (Ojo, 1970). According to these legends, first and foremost, Ile-Ife is the oldest and premier city of Yorubaland. Second, it is the center from which the dispersal of Yoruba settlements, culture, and tradition took place. Third, it is the only city of Yorubaland whose *Oba* (king), the *Ooni* of Ife, is the acknowledged spiritual ruler of the entire ethnic nation (Ojo, 1970). Though it has been very difficult to trace the dates of the founding of Ile-Ife, what is known indicates that it is an old settlement Biobaku. (1970) accounted for two waves of migrants from the northeast of the area. These cumulated in setting up of settlements in the 7th and 10th centuries around the land area of Ile-Ife. Similarly, Jefferys

Fig. 6: Map of Nigeria: Inset shows flag and position on a map of Africa.

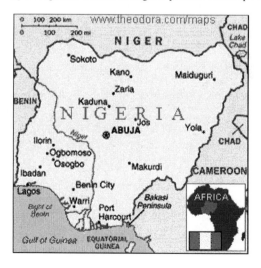

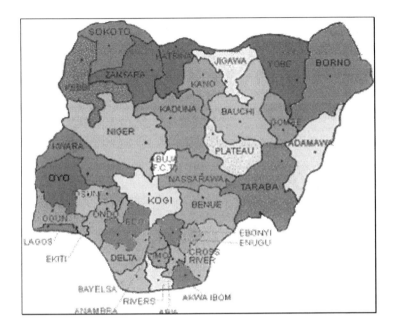

Fig. 7: The 36 states and Federal Capital Territory of Nigeria.

(1958) estimated that Ile-Ife became a flourishing city by the 11th century, shortly after the founding of Old Oyo, another important town in southwest Nigeria.

The original vegetation in the study area is of the equatorial tropical rainforest with its characteristic three-layer growth, evergreen, and luxuriant appearance all year round. This is being replaced by secondary rainforest, which is characterized by palm trees in most places. There are appearances of savanna type of vegetation with tall elephant grasses in parts that have been subjected to incessant use for farming (Adejuwon, 1979). Gallery types of forest are found along river valleys.

Annual average rainfall in the study area is about 200 centimeters with double maxima regime. Humidity is hardly below 80% all year round, while annual average temperature is usually high, between 24 and 27 degrees Celsius. There is a 3-month period of dry season with the prevalence of the harmattan wind reducing the temperature to the lowest in the year. The rock of the area is of the basement complex type, which is prevalent in the southwestern parts of the country (Iloeje, 1976). The soil, in most parts, is lateritic and clayey, with large deposits of laterite hard pans at the subsurface (Smith & Montgomery, 1965). However, the topsoil is rich in organic materials formed from the deposits and decay of vegetation (Iloeje, 1976).

The combination of climate type and good soil accounts for the extensive farming activities common among the people. Both the men and women are engaged in farming, either full time or a subsistence level (Iloeje, 1976). Since Ile-Ife is home to a university and two teaching hospitals, the people also engage in other different kinds of occupation other

21

than farming.

The Yorubas live in a contiguous environment. Because of the dichotomy in the structure of the urban and rural areas, subjects in the study were selected from both areas within the LGA.

Population and Sample

A previous study carried out by the Nigerian Association of Nurses and Nurse-Midwives (NANNM) placed FGM prevalence rate in Nigeria between 35% and 90% (WHO, 1996). According to the UNDS (1998), Osun State, with a rate of 98.7%, has the highest prevalence rate of FGM in Nigeria. The state was thus selected for this study because of its very high prevalence rate.

The sample population of the study was males and females of different ages residing in Ife East LGA of Osun State in Nigeria. The selection of respondents was based on stratification by geographical location (urban and rural). Questionnaires were administered to a total of 150 respondents in each of the urban and rural areas.

To select the respondents in the rural part of the LGA, the villages to be involved were first selected. The selection of the villages was based on past involvement in research work by the inhabitants. Most of the inhabitants of the selected villages had been involved with research conducted by the Department of Agricultural Extension and Rural Sociology of the Obafemi Awolowo University, Ile-Ife, Nigeria. The use of such people was necessary because of the sensitive nature of the research topic, which most of the people would rather not discuss. Therefore, the respondents needed to have a pre-fieldwork idea of what was going on. Their experience(s) in previous agricultural research provided this. Based on this point, the villages of Iyanfoworogi, Erefe, Laadin were selected. Fifty questionnaires were administered in each of the three villages, and with these, all the households in the villages were covered.

Urban respondents were selected from Oke-Ogbo and Ilode areas of the target LGA. All the households in Oke-Ogbo were involved, while for Ilode, respondents in the first 88 households who agreed to participate in the research were interviewed. In each of the households in both the rural and urban areas, according to the culture, the most elderly person present at the time, or somebody so designated, was interviewed.

In-depth interviews and focus group discussions were employed in collecting qualitative interviews for the study. The respondents of the questionnaire survey picked those involved in the in-depth interviews and for the focus group discussions. Discussants volunteered following invitations to take part in further group discussions on the topic.

Research Instruments

FGM is culture bound, and is reinforced by patriarchal attitudes and ideologies that are difficult to measure with standard survey techniques. Although quantitative data to measure incidence and prevalence rate were collected by means of an interview schedule, qualitative data were also collected through the use of in-depth interviews and focus group discussions, with the aid of pro-forma questions and a tape recorder. The need to balance the insider and outsider interpretations of the situation is very important to this type of culture-related sensitive research. The perspectives and the local definitions of the situation are gathered by listening to the people. In combining quantitative and qualitative measurement, therefore, an important weight was assigned to the respondents to document their beliefs and practices of FGM, and to suggest possible ways out of it as they considered it a problem. The insider/outsider perspective was considered because cultural groups tend to justify established practices. What is positive to the insider may be negative to the outsider.

Instruments used in collecting data were questionnaire interviews, in-depth interview of opinion leaders and of practitioners in the target communities, and focus group discussions. To develop the questions used in all the instruments, existing literature on the subject was reviewed, and key points to be investigated identified. Questions were then developed based on the points the research would want to investigate. The questions were pilot-tested twice. The first was in a private discussion involving the researcher and a small group of university lecturers in the Obafemi Awolowo Univeristy, Ile-Ife, Nigeria. The topic was brought up and the interview questions fielded. Also, during the first visit to the rural village heads, some of the questions were considered, after which a few of the questions were reviewed. The pilot tests also proved the necessity of the fieldwork being carried out the local language, since most of the respondents were more comfortable with in the Yoruba language.

The final draft of the questions was compared to the research objectives, and was seen to be adequate and appropriate. Please refer to Appendix A for the questionnaire and Appendix B for the set of questions utilized in the in-depth interviews and focus group discussions.

Data Collection Procedure

As part of the data collection procedure, a 2-day training exercise was carried out by the researcher and a female assistant, to train four women who were already experienced in conducting questionnaire interviews. During the training, the interview questions were considered in the local language, and the chances of ambiguity eliminated. The interview procedure was also standardized. Permission was requested and received from the heads of the rural communities involved in the research.

Quantitative data were collected with the interview schedule administered to 300 respondents. The questionnaire survey exercise took the four interviewers 10 days to complete, and the collection of qualitative data commenced after. This was executed by the researcher and his assistant. During the questionnaire survey, the respondents were asked to suggest opinion leaders who might be able to give further information on the topic. Based on their suggestions, those involved in the five in-depth interviews were picked. Two in-depth interviews of female opinion leaders were conducted, one in the rural and the other in the urban area. The village head in one of the rural villages, who also happened to be one of the oldest community members, was also interviewed. The other two in-depth interviews were with FGM practitioners, one in each of the urban and rural areas. All the interviews were conducted in the respondents' residence, and in the local language. They were all recorded on audiotapes.

Three focus group discussions were held. A female group discussion took place the in urban area. There were a total of 12 people, with 3 of them being under the age of 15 years. The discussion was held for about 1 hour 25 minutes. The two focus group discussions (male and female) in the rural area were conducted on the same day. While the male group had 7 men and was completed in about 1 hour 15 minutes, the female discussion lasted more than 2 hours. It was started with 8 women, but there were 12 by the time it was rounded up. Discussions were freely held with the prepared questions giving a general direction. Both discussions were recorded on audiotapes.

23

Analysis of Data

The quantitative collected data were analyzed using descriptive statistics such as frequency distribution, percentages, mean, standard deviation, and graphs.

The recorded in-depth interviews and focus group discussions were transcribed. The transcribed materials were analyzed for themes and categories, and were then used to provide added information and clarification to the structured interviews of the 300 rural and urban subjects.

CHAPTER FOUR

PRESENTATION OF RESULTS

This chapter presents and discusses the results of the data collected and analyzed. After discussing the demographic characteristics of the respondents, the responses are discussed according to the research questions as listed in chapter one.

Characteristics of respondents

As shown in Table 2, 46.3% of the respondents were above 40 years of age. About 24.0% were between 30 and 39 years old, 23.4% were between 20 and 29 years old, while 6.0% of the respondents were between 10 and 19 years old.

About 52.7% of the respondents, (Table 2), were female, while 47.3% were male; 72.0% were married, 20.0% were single, and 3.0% were divorced or widowed. Following the cultural pattern, a higher percentage (51.4%) of the married respondents were married into polygamous homes, and 32.9% had a monogamous marriage. A vast majority of the respondents (93.3%) belong to the Yoruba ethnic group, while 6.07% were Hausas, Igbos, or from some other tribes within Nigeria. Furthermore, 68.0% of the respondents were Christians, 29.7% were Muslims, and 2.0% practiced one form or another of traditional religion, while 0.3% practiced other unspecified forms of religion.

Level of Education

The data in Table 2 indicate that 30.3% of the respondents never had any form of formal education. Of the 17.4% that attempted primary school, 4.7% did not complete it. However, 6.3% and 30.3% completed Junior and Senior Secondary Schools, respectively. The other respondents were found at other levels of education, up to University-degree level. Analysis showed that just 69.7% of the respondents were literate, out of which 16.0% had at least one form of higher education.

Occupation

The distribution of the respondents spanned many vocations, as shown in Table 2. About 30.0% of them were farmers, 25.3% were traders, 12.7% were students, 11.7% were civil servants, 10.7% were professional artisans, and 8.3% were full-time housewives.

TABLE 2:

Distribution of Respondents according to Age, Gender, Marital Status, Type of Marriage, Ethnic group, Religion, Level of Education, and Occupation.

Age (years)	Frequency	Percentage	Marital Status	Frequency	Percentage
Less than 10	0	0.0	Single	60	20.0
10 to 19	18	6.0	Married	216	72.0
20 to 29	70	46.3	Divorced	3	1.0
30 to 39	72	23.4	Widowed	6	2.0
40 and above	139	46.3	No response	15	5.0
No response	1	0.3	**Total**	**300**	**100.0**
Total	**300**	**100.0**			
Gender	**Frequency**	**Percentage**	**Type of marriage**	**Frequency**	**Percentage**
Male	142	47.3	Polygamous	111	51.4
Female	157	52.3	Monogamous	71	32.9
No response	1	0.3	No response	34	15.7
Total	**300**	**100.0**	**Total**	**300**	**100.0**
Ethnic Group	**Frequency**	**Percentage**	**Religion**	**Frequency**	**Percentage**
Yoruba	280	93.3	Islam	89	29.7
Igbo	7	2.3	Christianity	204	68.0
Hausa	11	0.7	Traditional	6	2.0
Others	2	0.7	Others	1	0.3
Total	**300**	**100.0**	**Total**	**300**	**100.0**
Level of Education	**Frequency**	**Percentage**	**Occupation**	**Frequency**	**Percentage**
Did not go to school	91	30.3	Housewife	25	8.3
Did not complete primary education	14	4.7	Trading	76	25.3
Completed Primary School	38	12.7	Civil Servant	35	11.7
Junior Secondary School	19	6.3	Student	38	12.7
Senior Secondary School	90	30.0	Farming	90	30.0
Technical College	14	4.7	Professional	32	10.7
National Diploma	19	6.3	No response	4	1.3
University Degree	9	3.0	**Total**	**300**	**100.0**
Others (Adult literacy)	6	2.0			
Total	**300**	**100.0**			

Source: Author's research, March 2000

26

Research Question 1: What Are the Beliefs of the Respondents About Female Genital Mutilation (FGM)?

The respondents answered questions to ascertain their beliefs in the practice of Female Genital Mutilation in their area. There were eight such questions, and they included whether the respondents believed female children should be circumcised, and why; whether uncircumcised women should be allowed to get married, and why; if female children should be given a choice to get circumcised or not, and why; and the respondents' reactions where a daughter refuses to be circumcised. The questions were answered by choosing "yes" or "no" without a choice of "don't know."

FGM: To Be or Not to Be?

Analysis of collected data showed that the majority (70.0%) of the respondents believed that female children should be circumcised while 29.0% were against the practice. The remaining 1% did not respond to the question.

Many reasons were given by the respondents to substantiate their stand. On why it should be done, as seen on Table 3, 62.4% of the reasons were based on culture and ancient tradition. About 10.0% of the reasons were based on a continuity of what the elders had done. They declared it as a good act that should be continued. Another 8.1% said it is done to allay fear of future consequences, while 8.7% said it is done to prevent promiscuity in women. Only 2.8% of the reasons had a religious connotation, while 1.8 was based on health beliefs.

Of those who did not think females should be circumcised, 23.0% rejected it on health beliefs, and 16.1% of these specifically mentioned the possibility of contacting an infection from circumcision. Prominent among other reasons adduced against female circumcision are: the practice is rough, primitive, and annoying (17.2%); it shows disrespect for women (13.8%); campaigns from the media say it is not good (11.5%); and it deprives females of sexual enjoyment (10.3%).

FGM and Marriage

In the traditional Yoruba setting, marriage is an act that bestows a lot of respect on the woman. Therefore, the process of socialization amongst the Yorubas encourages that the crowning effect of growing up, for the female, is to be married. She is thus groomed to be physically, culturally, socially, and mentally fit for marriage.

Analysis of collected data showed that only 31.3% of the respondents agreed that uncircumcised women should be allowed to marry, while 67.0% were against allowing uncircumcised women to be married. Figure 8 indicate reasons why uncircumcised females should be, or should not be, allowed to marry.

Many of the respondents (32.7%) were against marriage of uncircumcised women because it is against their culture to permit such marriage. Based on information gathered from key informants who were interviewed and the participants

27

Position on Female Circumcision	Frequency	Percentage
YES to FGM	210	70.0
NO to FGM	87	29.0
No response	3	0.3
Total	**300**	**100.0**

Reasons for FGM	Frequency	Percentage
To allay fear of future consequences (bad events)	17	8.1
According to parents it is a good act	21	10.0
It is the culture as well as an ancient tradition	131	62.4
Uncircumcised clitoris can cause baby's death	10	4.8
It is a taboo/religious belief system	6	2.8
It controls promiscuity in women	18	8.7
It is good for health (prevents diseases)	4	1.8
Others	3	1.4
Total	**210**	**100.0**

Reasons against FGM	Frequency	Percentage
Disrespect to women folks	12	13.8
Rough, primitive and very annoying	15	17.2
Fear of infection	14	16.1
Dangerous to health	6	6.9
It is ungodly (no need for it)	2	2.3
Media campaign says it is not good	10	11.5
Deprive females of sexual enjoyment	9	10.3
Contradicts modern perception	7	8.1
Others	12	13.8
Total	**87**	**100.0**

Source: Author's research, March 2000

in the female focus group discussion, a woman who is uncircumcised is thereby being encouraged not to uphold tradition. Such a woman might remain deviant on some other cultural issues. While another 15.0% of the respondents also disagreed with such marriage because of unexplained health reasons, about 11.3% felt that marriage and circumcision are religious issues, and to be uncircumcised is a sign of unbelief. Another 4.7% believed that an uncircumcised female is promiscuous and will demand sex from her husband, which is a taboo and a sign of being flirtatious and having an uncontrolled sexual urge. Only 1.3% mentioned the safety of the baby during childbirth as their reason for being against marriage of uncircumcised women.

The strongest reason for allowing marriage of uncircumcised females include is the cultural importance of the marriage institution (15.7%). A small number (2.6%) would permit it because marriage of uncircumcised women is allowed in other cultures. Two percent also see it as a matter of choice of the woman and the groom.

Female Children's Choice on FGM

To elicit more information on the respondents' belief regarding female circumcision, they were asked if they believed that female children should have a choice in being circumcised. Data analysis showed that only 31.3% of the respondents felt that female children should have a choice on whether or not to be circumcised, while 68.7% were against giving the female child a choice.

As shown in Table 4, the most important reason for granting female children a choice was because 54.2% of those in support of this view considered Female Circumcision a human rights issue. If the child does not want to be circumcised, 23.9% reported this to be an acceptable reason. Some (8.5%) of the respondents declared that it is a cultural issue with no positive implication, while 7.0% felt it is no longer relevant. Another 6.4% believed it was against modern medical practice, as reproductive health issues in recent times are more concerned with females having a voice in matters that could impact their reproductive health life cycle.

A majority (62.1%) of those who believed children should not have a choice said it is the sole responsibility of parents to decide for their children on the issue of Female Circumcision. Another 27.7% said since it is carried out when the children are babies, they cannot have a choice anyway. Other reasons given include: children don't know the implication (1.9%), and uncircumcised women or their babies may die during childbirth later in life (0.5%). About 7.8% of those who carried this view did not give any reason.

It was generally agreed to in the focus group discussions and the point was also strongly presented in the key informant interviews that, in Yorubaland, parents always make decisions for their children until they are old enough and are married.

Reasons why respondents' are for or against marrying uncircumcised women

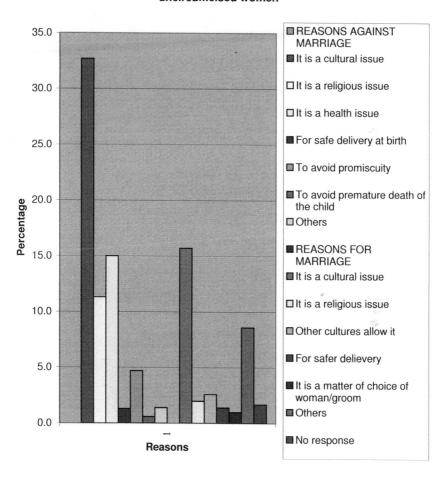

Source: Author's research, 2000

As shown in Table 4, the most important reason for granting female children a choice was because 54.2% of those in support of this view considered Female Circumcision a human rights issue. If the child does not want to be circumcised, 23.9% reported this to be an acceptable reason. Some (8.5%) of the respondents declared that it is a cultural issue with no positive implication, while 7.0% felt it is no longer relevant. Another 6.4% believed it was against modern medical practice, as reproductive health issues in recent times are more concerned with females having a voice in matters that could impact their reproductive health life cycle.

A majority (62.1%) of those who believed children should not have a choice said it is the sole responsibility of parents to decide for their children on the issue of Female Circumcision. Another 27.7% said since it is carried out when the children are babies, they cannot have a choice anyway. Other reasons given include: children don't know the implication (1.9%), and uncircumcised women or their babies may die during childbirth later in life (0.5%). About 7.8% of those who carried this view did not give any reason.

It was generally agreed to in the focus group discussions and the point was also strongly presented in the key informant interviews that, in Yorubaland, parents always make decisions for their children until they are old enough and are married.

Table 4:

Distribution of Respondent's according To Why It Should or Should Not Be Female Children's Choice to Get Circumcised

Position	Frequency	Percentage
Should be female children's choice	94	31.3
Should not be female children's choice	206	68.7
Total	**300**	**100**
Reasons for allowing children's choice	**Frequency**	**Percentage**
Some don't want it	34	23.9
It is a matter of right	77	54.2
It is a culture with no positive implication	12	8.5
Female circumcision is irrelevant today	10	7.0
Against modern medical development	9	6.4
Total	**142**	**100**
Reasons for allowing not children's choice	**Frequency**	**Percentage**
It is usually done at childhood	57	27.7
It is the sole responsibility of parents to decide	128	62.1
Children do not know the implications	4	1.9
She may die at child birth later	1	0.5
No specific reason	16	7.8
Total	**300**	**100**

Source: Author's research, March 2000

Reaction of Respondents to Refusal of Daughter and Spouse

The data in Table 5 show that the majority of the respondents (39.7% and 44.3%) would agree with their daughters who refused circumcision and spouse who refused circumcision for his or her daughter, respectively. Nearly the same proportion of respondents (36.3% and 37.0%) would use force on the daughter and spouse, respectively, to accept the mutilation, while a few respondents (22.7% and 14.7%) would allow time for deliberation over the issue.

Table 5

Reaction of Respondents to Refusal of Daughters and Spouse

Action on daughter who refuses circumcision	Frequency	Percentage
Agree with her	119	39.7
Force her to accept my way	109	36.3
Allow her to think over it	68	22.7
Others	4	1.3
Total	**300**	**100**
Action on spouse refusing circumcision of daughter	Frequency	Percentage
Agree with her/him	133	44.3
Disagree with her/him	111	37.0
Allow time to think over it	44	14.7
Others	12	4.0
Total	**300**	**100**

Source: Author's research, March 2000

Research Question 2: What Is The Level of the Respondents' Knowledge About FGM?

The respondents answered 10 knowledge-related questions in the questionnaire survey. These questions were in the area of the origin of Female Genital Mutilation, access to information concerning FGM, and the possibility of risks from the practice.

Knowledge of the Origin of FGM

Analysis of data collected indicated that very few of the respondents (7.7%) claimed to know the origin of FGM, while a vast majority (90.3%) had no knowledge of the origin of the practice. Of the possible origins suggested, 3.7% submitted that it is an age-long tradition practiced from ancient times. A small percentage of the respondent (2.0%) claimed that the practice must have originated from Yorubaland, while 0.3% said the origin could be found somewhere in the Bible and Quoran. About 94.0% of those who claimed knowledge of the origin of female circumcision could not substantiate their claim.

The origin of Female Genital Mutilation was not known by most of the study population. This was further validated by the conclusion of all those who were interviewed and those who participated in the focus group discussions.

General Information about FGM

A little over half (54.0%) of the respondents knew where to get necessary information on FGM, while the remaining 46% did not know. About 34.7% of the total population of respondents had sought information on FGM, while the large majority (65.3%) had never asked any question on the subject. It could be inferred that the majority of the respondents have not been seeking information on FGM because circumcision is a culturally accepted practice. Therefore it is not just a topic for normal or everyday discussion in the area.

Key informants who were interviewed attested to this point. It was also declared in

33

the male focus group discussion that only the mothers would want to acquire knowledge on FGM, since the only usual concern of the father was that it had to be carried out.

Risk at Birth to A Child Born of Circumcised Woman

Most of the respondents in the survey (81.7%) disagreed that children born to a circumcised woman are subject to risks at birth, while the remaining 16.0% believed that there are dangers for the baby and the circumcised mother during childbirth.

Adherents of the two positions gave a few reasons to support their views (Figures 9a – 9c). The three reasons advanced for the possibility of risks at birth are: excessive bleeding leading to death of mother or the child or both (66.7%), may result in still birth (8.3%), and problematic delivery because of perinea and genital tears (25%).

About 48.2% of the respondents believed that there could not be any risk to the child since the child's head will not touch the clitoris. Some (11.8%) believed there could not be any harm, while 4.1% of the respondents believed that the claim of any risk to the child of a circumcised mother is mere superstition. About 38.0% could not suggest any reason why they believed there was no risk to the baby.

Respondents' position on possibility of danger to child during childbirth if the mother is circumcised

Fig. 9a: Respondents' position

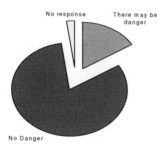

No response   There may be danger

No Danger

Fig. 9b: Reasons for the possibility of danger

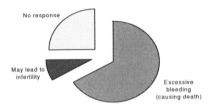

No response

May lead to
infertility

Excessive
bleeding
(causing death)

Fig. 9c: Reasons for no-danger position

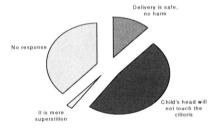

Delivery is safe,
no harm

No response

Child's head will
not touch the
clitoris

It is mere
superstition

Knowledge about Danger to Circumcised Women during Childbirth

Opinions again differ regarding whether circumcised women are faced with dangers during delivery of their babies. About 18.0% of the respondents believed that circumcised women face many dangers during delivery, while 82.0% said that circumcision does not cause women any problem during childbirth.

As seen in Table 6, 48.2% of those who said circumcised mothers face danger during childbirth have experienced "excessive bleeding" during childbirth and they believed it was caused by the circumcision. This is especially true for women who experienced Types II (excision) and III (infibulation), as corroborated during the focus group discussion and in-depth interviews. Other reasons given for holding on to this view were that delivery is painful (3.8%), and the pain is accompanied by restlessness (5.5%).

Of the respondents who took the position that circumcised mothers are not exposed to any danger at childbirth, 53.7% based their answer on experience, claiming that they never had any problem. Another 11.8% gave the same reason, claiming to have always delivered safely and easily. A similar reason was also given by another 14.1% who said circumcision ensured safe delivery, while 3.3% said it is safe because it had been going on for a long time.

Table 6:

Respondents' Knowledge about Danger to Circumcised Mother during Childbirth

Position	Frequency	Percentage
There are dangers to the circumcised mother	54	18.0
There is danger to the circumcised mother	246	82.0
Total	**300**	**100**
Reasons for Danger to circumcised mother	**Frequency**	**Percentage**
Parents impose on their daughters	5	9.3
Delivery is painful	3	3.8
Massive bleeding during childbirth	26	48.2
Possibility of experiencing tears	3	5.5
Causes terrible pain and restlessness	3	5.5
Others	12	22.2
No response	3	5.5
Total	**54**	**100.0**
Reasons for no danger to circumcised mother	**Frequency**	**Percentage**
Never a problem	132	53.7
Circumcised mother is free of any danger	8	3.3
I delivered my baby easily and safely	29	11.8
Should not entertain any fear	25	10.2
It gives safe delivery	35	14.1
It has been going on for a long time	8	3.3
Others	3	1.2
No response	6	2.4
Total	**246**	**100**

Source: Author's research, 2000

Knowledge about Transmission of Diseases during Circumcision

Respondents also shared different views and positions on the transmission of diseases during circumcision of female children. Despite the fact that 82% had earlier claimed that circumcised mothers are not prone to any danger at childbirth, about 61.3% of the respondents believed that diseases are usually and always transmitted during the operation. Some 38.7% of the respondents held to the view that no diseases are transmitted during female circumcision.

Many reasons were given in support of both positions (Table 7). Reasons given as to why diseases are transmitted after female circumcision are: diseases are transmitted during circumcision due to improper treatment of wounds (62.0%); application of local medicine (17.9%); use of unsterilized instruments (9.8%); contact with blood of diseased person (2.2%); no medication given after circumcision (3.3%); infertility resulting from infection (1.1%); and repeated use of same instrument for many children (1.6%).

In support of the position that no diseases are transmitted during and after circumcision, 20.7% simply said they had no record of transmission of diseases from female circumcision. Some said it is a usual practice, so the experts know how to carry out their job well (22.4%); there is no problem at childbirth or later in the future (6.9%) and clitoris cut-off

37

ensures that diseases are not harbored in the vagina (2.6%).

Table 7:

Distribution of Respondents According To Position on Whether Diseases Are Transmitted During FGM Operation or Not

Position	Frequency	Percentage
Diseases are transmitted	184	61.3
Diseases are not transmitted	116	38.7
Total	300	100
Reasons for transmission of disease	**Frequency**	**Percentage**
Improper treatment of wound	114	62.0
Use of local medicine	33	17.9
Use of unsterilized instruments	18	9.8
Contact with blood of diseased person	4	2.2
No medication given, causing infection	6	3.3
Infertility may result	2	1.1
Use of the same instrument for many children	3	1.6
Others	2	1.1
No response	2	1.1
Total	**184**	**100.0**
Reasons for None transmission of diseases	**Frequency**	**Percentage**
No disease can be transmitted	42	36.2
No record of disease transmitted	24	20.7
Experts know how well to do the job	26	23.4
Clitoris cut makes it safe	3	2.6
No problem during childbirth or later in life	8	6.9
Others	9	7.8
No response	4	3.4
Total	**116**	**100.0**

Source: Author's research, March 2000

The Practice of FGM in the Study Area

In order to collect information on the various aspects of FGM practice in the study area, respondents were asked to answer various questions. Discussions of the findings follow.

Research Question 3: What Are the Reasons for the Practice of FGM?

Data in Table 8 show the rank order of Mean Score on reasons for the practice of female circumcision, from the highest to the lowest. Tradition topped the rank with a 5.66 mean score, followed by enhanced fertility (2.67), and hygiene (2.63), while initiation came last with a mean score of 1.90.

The middle level reasons are preservation of virginity, pleasing husband, prevention of promiscuity, social acceptance, and health, with mean scores between 2.43 and 2.26. The lower level reasons are marriage-ability, peer group influence, and initiation.

From the in-depth interviews and female focus group discussions, the people generally believed that female circumcision was originally done to save the newborn baby from death. They believed that if the baby's head touched the clitoris during childbirth, the baby would die. However, according to the key informants, this belief is gradually fading because of modernization.

Table 8

Rank-Order of Mean Score of Reasons for FGM Practice

Reasons for Mutilation	Mean Score	Rank
Tradition	5.66	1st
Enhanced fertility	2.67	2nd
Hygiene	2.63	3rd
Preservation of virginity	2.43	4th
To please husband	2.34	5th
Prevention of promiscuity	2.30	6th
Social acceptance	2.27	7th
Health	2.26	8th
Sexual attraction	2.11	9th
Marriage-ability	2.09	10th
Peer group	2.00	11th
Initiation	1.90	12th

Source: Author's research, March 2000

Research Question 4: What is the Prevalence Rate of FGM in the Study Area?

Analysis of data collected during the study indicated that 57.0% of the female respondents were circumcised, 1.7% were not, while 41.3% did not respond. The non-response, according to some of the respondents, was due to the secrecy of the topic and that it is one they had never discussed before.

Information gathered from key informants indicated that virtually all females in the study area are circumcised. Status of the non-Yoruba women could not be evaluated. In the second female focus group discussion, 2 of the 12 participants had never heard of uncircumcised women.

Research Question 5: What Types of Circumcision Are Practiced?

Fig. 10 shows that Type 1 (clitoridectomy) is the most popular type of circumcision experienced by a majority of the female respondents (84.0%). This was followed by Type 2, which is called excision (15.20%). Just 1.0% of the respondents had experienced Type III (Infibulation).

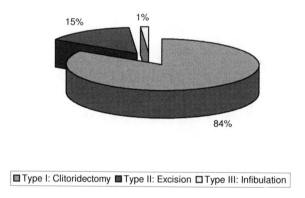

☐ Type I: Clitoridectomy ▨ Type II: Excision ☐ Type III: Infibulation

Fig. 10: Types of FGM in the study area.

Research Question 6: At What Age Is FGM Practiced in the Study Area?

Data in Figure 11 show that 41.0% of the respondents said that Female Genital Mutilation was carried out in the study area on the 8th day after childbirth. The participants of the female focus group discussion, who all agreed that it was usually performed on the 8th day, after the naming ceremony, corroborated this.

40

Few (11.3%) of the respondents claimed that it was done in their community between the ages of 1 and 5 years, while 3.0% said female circumcision age was between 5 and 20 years. According to the focus group discussion participants, those who experience the operation when matured might be from families where circumcision was usually celebrated or marked with the ability of the child to carry out a unique operation or activities for example, the ability to prepare pounded yam or a particular local soup or stew.

Key informants however claimed that where it was not performed before the age of 5, a young woman might have to be circumcised just before marriage or just before delivering her baby. While 2.3% did not know when the operation was usually performed, 42.3% did not respond to the question.

Fig 11: Age at which FGM operation is performed)

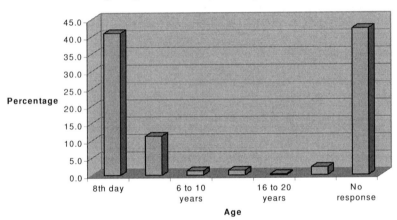

Regarding why circumcision is done at the age mentioned by the respondents, 54.3% again claimed tradition as the reason. Just 1.0% claimed a religious background, 0.3% said it is because of hygiene, while 44.4% of the respondents did not respond.

A reason agreed to by all the participants of the female focus group discussions is that female circumcision is done on the 8th day when the pain would be minimal, and because the painful effects would diminish faster at this period, than any other time in the child's life cycle.

Research Question 7: Who Are the Practitioners of FGM in the Study Area?

Data in Table 9 show the practitioners of FGM in the study area in order of frequency distribution. Local circumciser (*Olola*), is ranked first at 49.8%, followed by Trained Nurse (3.7%), Traditional Birth Attendants (TBA) (2.3%), Medical Doctor (2.0%), Barber (1.3%),

41

and Native Doctor (1.0%). About 40.3% of the respondents did not respond. These are probably males since the mothers take the children for circumcision in the study area.

Key informant interviews with a male opinion leader, two women, and two practitioners gave further information. Up till about 1995, the local circumciser who is called *Olola,* in the local language, performed all the operations. However, in the last few years, Community Health Workers, Traditional Birth Attendants, and, in some cases, trained nurses, have taken over the job. Both practitioners interviewed said an average of four operations were performed per month in their respective communities. For both of them, circumcision was the family business, which they inherited from their fathers. However, they both had apprentices who were undergoing training in order to acquire the skill of performing male and female circumcision.

The local practitioners in the study area usually have other vocations, the most prominent of which is farming.

Table 9

Rank-Order of Practitioners of FGM Based On Frequency Distribution

Type of Practitioner	Frequency	Percentage
Local Circumcisor *(Olola)*	148	49.8
Trained Nurse	11	3.7
Traditional Birth Attendant (TBA)	7	2.3
Medical Doctor	6	2.0
Barber	4	1.3
Native Doctor	3	1.0
No response	121	40.3
Total	**300**	**100.0**

Source: Author's research, March 2000

Research Question 8: How Are the Practitioners Paid?

Findings showed that there is no fixed amount in monetary term or specific items in material term, granted practitioners as payment for the job done.

Data in Table 10 showed that money and/or items given out by parents to practitioners in exchange for each circumcision range from nothing to some amount of money, a maximum of which is less than N600.00 ($6.00). About 21.2% of the respondents said between N10.00 (10 cents) and N100 ($1.00) is given to the practitioner. Some (11.4%) claimed items like snails and kolanuts of no specific quantity are given without any monetary reward; 10.7% said less than 10 cents is given, while 3.7% would not give anything for the operation in the study area. In one of the villages in which the study was conducted, the official price per operation was put at N150 ($1.50). Mothers could also give up to three large tubers of yam for the circumcision of their daughters. Obviously the remuneration of practitioners varies from community to community in the study area.

Table 10:

Remuneration Paid To Practitioners for Each Circumcision Operation

Remuneration	Frequency	Percentage
Nothing	11	3.7
Snail and/ or kolanut	34	11.4
Token amount (below 10 cents)	32	10.7
Between 10 cents and $1	63	21.2
Between $1 and $2	12	4.0
Between $2 and $3	11	3.6
Between $3 and $4	3	1.0
Between $4 and $5	0	0.0
Between $5 and $6	1	0.3
No response	130	43.8
Total	**300**	**100.0**

Source: Author's research, March 2000

Research Question 9: What Instruments Are Used in the Operation?

As shown in Fig. 12, many types of instruments were used for female circumcision in the study area. These include knife (4.0%), pair of scissors (41.7%), and razor blade (5.7%). To substantiate this, information was collected from key informants, who included two practitioners. They claimed to utilize pairs of scissors most of the time and a razor blade some of the time. Care of instruments depended on the type of instrument used and the practitioner. For the local practitioner, once used, the pair of scissors or the razor blade is usually washed with water and kept in a safe place (like the inside of a bag hanging on the wall) in readiness for the next operation.

About 40% of the respondents did not react to this question. These are most likely men who do not usually get directly involved with the operation.

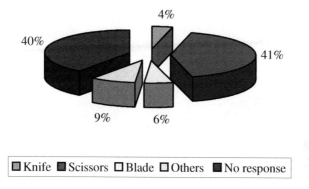

4%

40%

41%

9%   6%

| Knife | Scissors | Blade | Others | No response |

Fig. 12: Instruments used for FGM Operations in the study area.

Research Question 10: What Post-operation Cares Are Given?

As seen in the data in Fig. 13, items used for post-FGM operation care include herbs (37.0%), first-aid materials (14.3%), and other items (7.3%). Many of the respondents (40.6%) did not respond. This is probably because the men do not usually witness the operation and so could not have known the immediate treatment given. In the interviews conducted, the practitioners declared during the interviews that different types of local herbs were used to stop the bleeding and to reduce pain. In the women focus group discussion, it was also revealed that the first-aid given was usually analgesic to reduce pain, and some other drugs to reduce fever that may develop. Such drugs are given mainly by nurses and TBA.

Fig. 13: FGM Post-Operation care in the study area

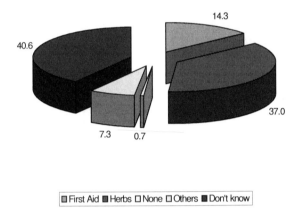

14.3

40.6

37.0

7.3   0.7

☐ First Aid ▨ Herbs ☐ None ☐ Others ■ Don't know

Research Question 11: What Are the Post-operation Complications?

Generally, there are two groups of FGM post-operation complications. These are the immediate and the long-term complications.

The major immediate post-operation complications in the study area were: urinary retention (25.7%), pain (9.7%), and infection/fever (4.7%). The less frequent ones are hemorrhage (2.3%), shock (2.0%), and pain (1.0%). About 14.3% of the respondents said there were no immediate complications, while 40.3% did not respond.

Mothers who participated in the focus group discussion declared that pain felt by the baby is the most obvious immediate post-operation effect. The babies also cry a lot the first time they urinate after the operation. Although subsequent urinations would not be as painful, the urine is usually retained until the baby can not bear it any longer.

In terms of the long-term effects, 46.7% of the respondents said there were none, and another 46.0% claimed they did not know. In addition, 4.0% had experienced prolonged labor due to the operation. Other long-term complications were the development of cysts (0.3%) and frigidity (1.3%).

During the female focus group discussion, it was discovered that some of the respondents usually hide the effects of their circumcision, or their daughter's circumcision, from the public. In reaction to the silence that first followed the question asked to find out the effects of FGM, one of the women declared: "Most people, fathers and mothers, would

45

not confess that circumcision caused problems for them or their babies. They usually tie the problem to other causes." Most of the participants agreed with her.

Table 11

Post-Operation Complications Experienced in the Study Area

Immediate complication	Frequency	Percentage
Hemorrhage	7	2.3
Shock	6	2.0
Infection (fever)	14	4.7
Urinary retention	77	25.7
Pain	29	9.7
None	45	14.3
Don't know	122	40.3
Total	**300**	**100.0**
Long-term complication	**Frequency**	**Percentage**
Cyst	1	0.3
Frigidity	4	1.3
Infertility due to infection	4	1.3
Prolonged obstructed labor	12	4.0
Tears	1	0.3
None	140	46.7
Don't know	138	46.0
Total	**300**	**100.0**

Source: Author's research, March 2000

Research Question 12: What Is the Attitude of Men About Marriage to Uncircumcised Women?

Analysis of data collected showed that 42.3% of the male respondents married or might marry an uncircumcised woman, while 57.7% chose not to marry an uncircumcised woman.

Some of the data in Table 12 show that respondents will not marry an uncircumcised woman for many reasons such as: culture/tradition reasons (73.2%), sexual reasons (1.2%), and religious reasons (12.2%). Other reasons include: non-acceptability by peer group (3.6%) and fear of promiscuity (6.2%). About 3.6% took the step without any specific reason. The village head who was interviewed declared that he would not have a relationship with an uncircumcised woman. He felt it was inconceivable. When pressed for a specific reason, he gave a cultural and traditional one.

Reasons why some of the respondents will marry an uncircumcised woman include: embrace new system and forget the old idea (13.3%), nothing bad in marrying an uncircumcised woman (6.7%), personal interest (23.5%), to avoid transmission of STD and AIDS diseases (10.0%), to change sexual style (31.7%), uncircumcised women are sensitive to sex (10.0%), and avoidance of problems during childbirth (5.0%).

46

Table 12:

Distribution of Male Respondents According To Decision to Marry or Not To Marry Uncircumcised Women

Position	Frequency	Percentage
To marry	60	42.3
Not to marry	82	57.7
Total	**142**	**100**
Reasons against	**Frequency**	**Percentage**
Religious reason	10	12.2
Cultural reason	60	73.2
Sexual reason	1	1.2
Unacceptable to peer group	3	3.6
Fear of promiscuity	5	6.2
No specific reason	3	3.6
Total	**82**	**100.0**
Reasons for	**Frequency**	**Percentage**
Embrace new system, forget the old idea	8	13.3
Nothing bad in marrying uncircumcised woman	4	6.7
Personal interest	14	23.3
Avoid transmission of STD and AIDS	6	10.0
To change sexual	19	31.7
Uncircumcised women are more sensitive	6	10.0
To avoid problem at childbirth	3	5.0
Total	**60**	**100.0**

Source: Author's research, March 2000

Research Question 13: What Are the Effects of FGM on Men?

An analysis of findings during the survey showed that the majority of the respondents (69.2%) will circumcise their daughters, while 29.1% said they would not.

Findings from the interviews and focus group discussions conducted indicated that some men would divorce their wife if they discovered that she was not circumcised, or if the wife refused to circumcise their daughter. Most of these men were over 45 years of age. They claimed the father sees circumcision as a sign of ownership of the child.

The older men who took part in the male focus group discussion agreed that if Female Genital Mutilation is meant to curb promiscuity, then the women are meant not to derive any enjoyment in sexual relations. Some of these men concluded that since some of them give this as a reason for marrying more wives, then Female Genital Mutilation must be contributing to promiscuity among men, and also encouraging polygamy.

This point will need to be studied further before a conclusion can be reached.

47

Research Question 14: What Is the Attitude of the People Toward Modification and Elimination of FGM in Their Community?

Nearly 50% of the respondents (48.7%) agreed to a modification of the practice, 37.0% were against it, while 14.3% did not respond. However, further questioning showed that just 4.7% of the respondents supported modification of the type of circumcision for female children, 29.3% advocated modification on the operator, while 6.7% supported modification in relation to instrument used and post-operative treatments given.

Regarding whether the practice of Female Genital Mutilation should be discontinued or not, analysis of findings showed that the majority of the respondents (66.0%) wanted the practice to continue unabated, 31.3% wanted a it stopped, while 2.4% did not respond.

From these findings, it could be deduced that FGM is still popular in the study area and that it will take some time and effort to put a stop to it.

Reasons For and Against Stoppage of FGM Practice

Data in Table 13 show the reasons for and against eliminating Female Genital Mutilation in the study area. About 13.4% of the respondents wanted it stopped because of its harmful nature to the child, 9.0% saw it as a barbaric act, which is no longer necessary, and because of some difficulties it had caused during childbirth (6.7%).

The major reasons against stopping FGM in Ife East Local Government of Osun State, Nigeria, are also three in number. About 31.7% of the respondents are of the view that it is a traditional act and tradition should not be stopped, 20.3% felt it is a matter of choice; therefore the government should not force any family to stop it. And 7.7% claimed that it is not injurious to anybody, not even the child, therefore, it should not be stopped. Only 2.3% felt that stopping FGM would increase promiscuity among females.

The findings indicated that without cultural sustainability efforts, it might be easy to stop Female Genital Mutilation.

Table 13:
Distribution of Respondents According To Reasons Why FGM Should or Should Not Be Stopped

Reasons why FGM should be stopped	Frequency	Percentage
It is harmful to children	40	13.3
It is a painful practice	8	2.7
Doctor's advise	7	2.3
No longer necessary (it is barbaric)	27	9.0
Difficulty at childbirth	20	6.7
Reasons why FGM should be stopped	**Frequency**	**Percentage**
It can't be stopped, it is a matter of choice	61	20.3
It is not injurious to anybody	23	7.7
Our tradition must not be stopped	95	31.7
To prevent promiscuity	11	3.7
No response	8	2.7
Total	**300**	**100.0**

Source: Author's research, March 2000

48

Summary

Female Genital Mutilation (FGM) is one of the traditional practices with recognized negative social, health, and psychological side effects. Unfortunately, sexuality as a topic is not discussed in many African societies. The silence over the topic has created a lack of information about FGM, helping to sustain the practice, and deceiving women to play an active role in upholding it.

This study examined the practice among a group reported to have a prevalence rate of more than 98%. It is expected to contribute information on the knowledge, belief, and practice of FGM among this group, which will form a basis for the development of culturally appropriate plans to eliminate the practice.

About 53% of the respondents were females, 72% were married into mainly polygamous homes, 93% were Yorubas, 68% were Christians, and about 29% were Muslims. Nearly 70% of the respondents had had one form of formal education or the other. Most of them were farmers and traders, with another 25% being full-time housewives.

The majority of the respondents (70%) believed the female children should be circumcised and the practice should continue unabated. The major reasons adduced were culture and ancient tradition, and to save babies from death as their heads touch the mothers' uncircumcised clitoris at childbirth. However, there were some of the respondents who did not agree with the practice because they saw it as "rough, primitive and annoying" and one that "shows disrespect for the female gender." A few were against FGM for health reasons.

No specific origin could be identified for the practice in the area, except that it has been a long-time tradition. The self-reported prevalence rate was 57%, though more than 40% of the women declined to answer the question. The two most common types of FGM were Types I (84%) and II (15%), which resulted in pain and urinary retention. Another post-operation complication was infection that may lead to infertility of the woman. Local practitioners (*Oloola*), Traditional Birth Attendants, trained nurses, and medical doctors were practitioners of FGM. They make use of scissors and blades to carry out their operations. The wounds were treated with local herbs and other materials.

About 58% of the men reported they would not marry an uncircumcised woman, while 67% of all the respondents believed marriage of uncircumcised women should not be permitted, to keep up the tradition. In the male focus group discussion session, a possible link between FGM and polygamy was identified. Despite this, 66% of the respondents did not want the practice stopped, while 48.7% advocated for a modification.

49

CHAPTER FIVE

DISCUSSION, CONCLUSION, AND RECOMMENDATIONS

Discussion

A reason widely reported in existing literature (Kopelman, 1994; WHO 1996, 1997) was also declared by a majority of the respondents in the research, as the basis for practice of FGM in the study area. FGM is a practice based on culture and tradition. This is what makes the eradication of the practice difficult, because the underlying cultural values will be difficult to disregard. This difficulty stems from the fact that the moral judgment from one culture may not have any relevance to what is right or wrong in another culture. After all, according to some versions of ethical relativism, if an issue is approved in a culture, then it is right if practiced in that culture (Kopelman, 1994). That is why any program put in place to tackle the problem of FGM must take the people's culture into consideration.

The reasons given by the 29% who rejected FGM showed the effects of Western education, media campaigns, and modernization. Some of the people in this group actually declared the practice to be against the advice given in the media. A few (8.1%) declared it as being against modern perceptions. Western education has obviously made a mark, but as advocated by Okunade (1997), an aggressive pursuit of female education, that the people will see to have taken the local culture into consideration, will further raise the people's awareness on the subject.

Despite the importance of marriage in the culture of the Yorubas, 67% would prefer uncircumcised women staying unmarried for life if they do not succumb to mutilation. Of all the respondents, 32.7% took this position to uphold the culture. Ironically, another 15.7% of the respondents supported marriage of uncircumcised women also for cultural reasons, indicating the importance of marriage to the Yoruba woman. This shows that while cultural practices differ from tribe to tribe, interpretation of cultural acts may be different even within each ethnic group.

The Yoruba culture gives the parents full responsibility for their children, and, in some households, the control continues even after the children are married. This explains why 68.7% of the respondents thought it was unspeakable for decisions concerning FGM to be left with the children. While most of the respondents in this group must have been adults, those who took the other view were the younger ones who felt it was their right to decide because some of them just "don't want it."

The people were not well informed about the practice of FGM. The basic reason for this was because the topic of sexuality is one that is hardly discussed, as also mentioned by those interviewed and in all the focus group discussions. Therefore, 65.3% of the respondents declared they had never discussed the topic, an indicator of the conservative nature of the people on the subject of sexuality. Efforts are already being made to include sex education in school curriculums. If successful, this might help diffuse some of the mysteries surrounding the subject.

It was reported by 81.7% that there were no risks at all to the child of a circumcised woman during childbirth, and by 82% that the mother herself faced no danger. This would

50

not be true in communities where Types II and III are practiced. But the Type I practiced in the study area reduces the immediate effects of FGM to mainly infection, as agreed to by about 61.3% of the respondents who reported that diseases were transmitted during operation. Such infections emanated from "improper treatment of wounds", "use of local medicine", and the "use of unsterilized instruments." Herbs are important among the Yorubas in treating all types of ailments. Traditional doctors, who have been given recognition in the society use leaves, stems, and roots to treat even the most complicated diseases. This indicates again that other solutions will have to be looked into, because the use of herbs cannot be stopped in Yorubaland.

The research showed a self-reported prevalence rate of 57%, although 41.3% of the female respondents did not respond. Some were surprised and obviously embarrassed that such questions were being asked. However, information gathered from the two focus group discussions indicated that virtually all women in the study area were circumcised. If it is assumed that the 41.3% who did not respond were circumcised, as declared by the focus group discussion participants, this would bring the prevalence rate to 98.3%, which agrees with to the 98.7% reported by the UNDS (1998) study.

The FGM operation is carried out mainly on the 8th day in the study area, indicating a link with the biblical injunction of circumcision of male children on the 8th day. Against medical ethics, more and more trained medical personnel were becoming involved with the FGM operations. As far as the local practitioners interviewed were concerned, putting a stop to the practice would not have an adverse effect on them because the income from the practice was low and they had their farms and sale of herbs to fall back on. While some writers such as Jacobs (1993) feel the resistance against FGM elimination is most likely to come from the local practitioners who will be losing a source of livelihood, such resistance in the study area may be from the trained nurses who seem to have discovered a source of extra income.

The results of the research show that both men and women were influential to the continuation of the practice. Of the men, 57.7% declared they would not marry an uncircumcised woman, mainly for cultural reasons. However, as declared in the male focus group discussion session, most of them would not even know if their wives were circumcised or not. Proceedings of the male focus group discussions indicated that only the very old men are against changing the status quo. The younger generation of men seems ready to do away with the FGM practice. It seems, over time, an increasing number of men would turn against the practice. If future education programs on the subject will take this into consideration, it is likely that the women who carry their daughters and granddaughters to the practitioners for the operation will re-think their position.

Both FGM and polygamy are practices entrenched in the Yoruba culture. The possible connection identified between them during the male focus group discussion will need further study.

The men were more ignorant than the women in that the men did not respond to many questions because, as reported, they did not know. The men knew enough however, to conclude at the male focus group discussion session that FGM was likely to be encouraging polygamy among the people if it is true that the practice reduces sexual enjoyment for the women.

Since the practice was based on tradition, 66% wanted it to continue, while 31.3% wanted a stop to it. Nearly half of the respondents declared that if it must continue, modification of one or all of the practitioners, instruments, and post-operation care will be

51

necessary. It is a positive development that the people wanted a modification because it reveals that they saw something wrong with the practice. However, the modification of practitioners, which may permit trained medical personnel to operate, will be counter-productive in that the practice may then become more difficult to stop.

Conclusion

FGM is so entrenched in the culture and ways of life of the people in the study area that the majority of those who claimed to have knowledge of it reported they do not see the harmfulness of the practice. Therefore it is not surprising that there were parents who still would enforce it on their female children. The fact that the victims of FGM in this area were not visibly complaining, as they are victims of a practice to which they are voluntarily submitted to (by parents), explains the continuity and perpetuation of the practice. Most of the reasons adduced for performing FGM operations are glaringly based on the status of women dependent on their marriage-ability and lack of knowledge about its health consequences. These led the women to accept the practice in the name of tradition and culture. The use of the term "Circumcision" rather than "Female Genital Mutilation," and the thought by some that it is religiously founded, continue to continue to perpetuate misinformation, in the Yoruba culture, in this instance. The response of the people in the study area portrays FGM more as an acquired idea or practice, which in a simplified and demystified form has no legal ideologies to justify it.

It is not in all instances that tradition is immutable and must remain constant.
It is quite agreeable that there is need for continuity and preservation of cultural heritage. This custom performs no useful purpose, and yet is epidemiologically harmful, and visibly seen to connote harm to the practicing communities. Adjustments and changes that will address cultural values and allow for developmental benefits will be rewarding.

Recommendations

The complexity of the practice of FGM, its prevalence, severity, and the wide variety in its social rationale within a sub-region, or large country like Nigeria, calls for the need to involve the grass-roots organization and principal stakeholders in leading the way to eradicate or discontinue its practice. A lot is still to be done if women in this area are to realize the harmful effects of FGM. The impact of the NANNM in Nigeria in keeping FGM in the focus of the media has yielded fruits in creating awareness. As the respondents in both this study and that of the UNDS (1998) report showed, quite a number of people learned about the negative consequences of FGM through the media, thus creating awareness. There is however the need to go beyond the awareness level, if change is going to be imparted. There is a need to suggest strategies to mobilize the people so that positive change may happen.

For instance, there is the need to educate female and male opinion leaders, parents, and female and male adolescents about the harmfulness of FGM operations. Putting it on the State and National agenda will help to remove the secrecy and obscurity surrounding it. Such discussions should involve opinion leaders. An effective education campaign would debunk the fact that discussion on FGM is a sign
of lack of control of sexual urge or waywardness. Other West African countries such as Ghana and Burkina Faso (Population Reference Bureau, 1996) have implemented initiatives to provide other employment for practitioners, so that their opposition to change will be reduced. The ones in this study area are already engaged in farming. They could be encouraged with the grant of soft loans and fertilizers, among others. This is because

intervention efforts by Inter-African Committee (IAC) in the southwestern part of Nigeria, which includes the study area, showed that practitioners usually oppose intervention programs, as such programs are seen by them as a means of depriving them of their source of livelihood and position within the society (IAC, 1999). If given the opportunity of seeing their alternative occupation as being lucrative, sustaining, and sustainable, they might reduce opposition and relinquish their 'exalted' positions of circumcisers. Also, alternative provision of jobs should be created for practitioners who do not have an alternative source of livelihood. They could be trained and equipped for other vocations such as shoe repair work, tailors, etc., along with training programs that will educate them on the sexual and psycho-social harmfulness of FGM. Trained medical personnel who are getting involved in the practice will have to be strongly discouraged.

Education programs that will sensitize and consciousness-raise women leaders and women groups could be exploited, with real-life case studies on the accompanying harmful consequences of FGM. These are likely to bring the need for positive steps toward elimination of the practice into the focus of the women.

Though the 1999 International Conference on Population and Development (IAPD) held in Cairo recommended legislative change to FGM by asking governments to prohibit FGM wherever it exists, and give vigorous support to efforts among NGO, CBOs, and religious institutions, to eliminate the practice, laws are not
likely to end or eliminate FGM. Although this would show government's commitment to its elimination, it could lead to a tussle between the citizenry and government such as what happened in Egypt, which eventually led to the reversal of the 35-year ban of FGM in government hospitals in Egypt (Kiragu, 1995).

In Nigeria today, under the democratic rule, only the Edo State government has given a government commitment to FGM elimination through its legislative body: the Edo State House of Assembly. It is, however, too early to ascertain the effect of this legislation of FGM. Legislative change will, however, not be recommended in this case as it is not participatory and therefore will only be addressing the problem in isolation of its stakeholders. Also, legislation is likely to increase the secrecy surrounding FGM practice, and the indication of a penalty will only drag the practitioners underground and make them less visible. This, of course, will only make the consequences more difficult to treat and control.

Since FGM practice has developmental connotations, further examination of the role of the women whose welfare is at stake is needed. Their empowerment and use of their personal relationship within their societies are needed to effect the required change. Further appraisal of the role of FGM in encouraging polygamy and the spread and prevalence of AIDS where FGM is practiced is also needed.

BIBLIOGRAPHY

Abdalla, R. H. D. (1982). *Sisters in affliction: Circumcision and infibulation in Africa*. London: Zed Press.

Abusharaf, R. M. (1998). Unmasking tradition: A Sudanese anthropologist confronts female 'circumcision' and its terrible tenacity. *The Sciences, 38*, 22-27.

Abusharaf, R. M. (2000, March). Female circumcision goes beyond feminism. *Anthropology News*, 17, 18.

Adejuwon, J. O. (1979). *An introduction to the geography of the tropics*. Lagos: Nelson.

Action Health Incorporated. (1997, March). FGM is a violation of girls' rights. *Growing Up: A Newsletter for Young People*, 2.

Adebajo, C. O. (1992). Female circumcision and other dangerous practices to women's health. In M. K. Kisekka (Ed.), *Women's health issues in Nigeria*. Zaria, Nigeria: Tamaza Publishing Company.

Akinyele-George, Y. (1997). Nigerian law and female circumcision. In B. E. Owumi (Ed.), *Primary health care in Nigeria: Female circumcision* (pp. 5:20-24). Ibadan: Cadalad Nigeria.

Althaus, F. A. (1997). Female circumcision: Rite of passage or violation of rights. *International Family Planning Perspectives, 23*(3), 1-6.

Baasher, T. A. (1979). *Psychological aspects to female circumcision*. Proceedings of the WHO Seminar on Traditional Practices Affecting the Health of Women and Children, Khartoum, Sudan.

Badri, A. E. (1972). Female circumcision in the Sudan: Change and continuity. In *Women and Reproduction in Africa* (Occasional Paper Series, no. 5). Dakar: AFARD-AAWORD.

Badri, G. (1979). *The views of gynecologists, midwives and college students on female circumcision*. Proceedings of the Symposium on the Changing Status of Sudanese Women, Ahfad University College for Women, Omdurman, Sudan.

Badri, S. (1983). *Knowledge and attitudes toward female circumcision by high school girls*. Omdurman, Sudan: Ahfad University College for Women.

Biobaku, S. O. (1970). *The origin of the Yoruba* (Monograph Series No. 1). Lagos: University of Lagos.

Center for Gender and Social Policy Studies. (1999). *An overview of gender discrimination and harmful traditional practices in Nigeria.* Unpublished manuscript, Obafemi Awolowo University, Ile-Ife, Nigeria.

Chelala, C. (1998, July 11). An alternative way to stop female genital mutilation. *Lancet, 352*(9122), 126.

Dorkenoo, E. E. (1992). *Female genital mutilation: Proposal for change.* London: Minority Group International.

Dorkenoo, E. (1994). *Cutting the rose: Female Genital Mutilation; the practice and its prevalence.* London: Minority Group International.

Ebomoyi, E. (1987). Prevalence of female circumcision in Nigeria communities. *Sex Roles, 17,* 3-4.

El Dareer, A. (1982). *Women, why do you weep? Circumcision and its consequences.* London: Zed Press.

Federal Government of Nigeria. (1989). *The constitution of the Federal Republic of Nigeria.* Lagos: Federal Government Press.

Hendsbee, M. (1998). *What's missing? A look into Female Genital Mutilation.* Unpublished manuscript.

Hetata, S. (1997). *Nawal El Saadawi: The hidden face of Eve.* London: Zed Books.

Hosken, F. P. (1979). The Hosken Report: Genital and sexual mutilation of females. *Women's International Network News,* vol., issue, page.

Iloeje, N. P. (1976). *A new geography of Nigeria.* Ibadan: Longman Nigeria.

Institute for Development Training. (1993, Summer). Female Genital Mutilation-- Initiatives for prevention. *Women's International Network News, 19*(3), 44.

Inter-African Committee on Traditional Practices. (1990, November). *Short activity reports from IAC counterparts in Africa for the period 1987-1990.* Prepared for the IAC Conference in Addis Ababa, Ethiopia.
Inter-African Committee on Traditional Practices. (1999). Manuscript presented at UNICEF-organized FGM workshop for NGOs and CBOs in Zone B, Southwest Nigeria.

Jacobs, G. (1993). *Female Genital Mutilation.* N.p.: Edna McConnel Clack Foundation.

Jefferys, M. D. (1958). When Ile-Ife was founded. *Nigeria Field, 23*(1).

Kiragu, K. (1995). *Female Genital Mutilation: A reproductive concern.* Supplements to Population Reports, Meeting the Needs of Young Adults. Baltimore: John Hopkins Center for Communication Programs.

Kopelman, L. M. (1994, October). Female circumcision/genital mutilation and ethical relativism. *Second Opinion, 20*(2), 55-71.

Koso-Thomas, O. (1987). *The circumcision of women: A strategy for eradication.* London: Zed Books.

National Committee on Traditional Practices in Ethiopia. (1995, Winter). AIDS and Female Genital Mutilation. *Women's International Network News, 21*(1), 34.

Negerie, M. (1997). *Position paper on Female Genital Mutilation.* Report presented to the ADRA International Board of Trustees, Washington, DC.

Ojo, A. (1970). Some aspects of the historical and cultural geography of Ife. In S. A. Agboola (Ed.), *The Ife regions.* Ibadan: University Press.

Oke, E. A. (1997). "Tradition versus modernity: The issue of female circumcision." In B. E. Owumi (Ed.), *Primary health care in Nigeria: Female circumcision* (pp. 4:15-19). Ibadan: Cadalad Nigeria.

Okunade, A. (1997). Health implications of Female Genital Mutilation. In B. E. Owumi (Ed.), *Primary health care in Nigeria: Female circumcision* (pp. 3:9-14). Ibadan: Cadalad Nigeria.

Osun State of Nigeria Ministry of Health, Vaccine Cold Chain Office. (1999). *Target population for 1999 30LGAs.* Osogbo, Nigeria: Author.

Owumi, B. E. (1993). *A socio-cultural analysis of female circumcision among the Urhobos: Study of the Okpe people of Delta State.* A monograph submitted to Inter African Committeee on Traditional Practices Affecting the Health of Women and Children in Nigeria.

Owumi, B. E. (1994). Forms and age of circumcision: Some psychological implications for women's fertility. *Journal of Women's Behavioral Issues, 1*(1), 2-4.

Owumi, B. E. (1997). Forms of circumcision and its implications for the women folk. In B. E. Owumi (Ed.), *Primary health care in Nigeria: Female circumcision* (pp. 2-8). Ibadan: Cadalad Nigeria.

Population Reference Bureau. (1996). T*he world's youth 1996.*

Public Health Reports. (1998). UN agencies join against FGM/FC. *Public Health Report, 113*(1), 6.

Rushwan, H. (1990, April-May). Female circumcision. *World Health*, 24-25.

Saleh, A. B. (1982). Circumcision and infibulation in the Sudan: Traditional practices affecting the health of women and children. *Journal of Women's Behavioral Issues, 1*(1), page.

Sarau, A. R. (1998, April). Turning up the volume of our sisters' voices. *Essence, 28*(12), 172.

Smith, A. S., & Montgomery, R. F. (1965). *Soils and land use in Central Western Nigeria.* Ibadan: Government Printers.

Toubia, N. (1995). Female Genital Mutilation: A call for global action. New York: Women Ink.

United Nations Development System (1998). *National baseline survey of harmful and positive traditional practices affecting women and girls in Nigeria.* A report submitted to UNDS, Lagos, by the Center for Gender and Social Policy Studies, Obafemi Awolowo University, Ile-ife, Nigeria.

World Health Organization. (1986). A traditional practice that threatens health Female circumcision. *WHO Chronicle, 40*(1), 31-36.

World Health Organization. (1996). WHO *information kit.* Geneva: Author.

World Health Organization. (1997). *Female Genital Mutilation: A joint WHO/UNICEF/UNFPA statement.* Geneva: Author.

World Bank. (1994). Better *health in Africa: Experience and lessons learned.* Washington, DC: World Bank Publication.

Women's International Network. (1993, Winter). AIDS Training Program: The eradication of Female Genital Mutilation. *Women's International Network News, 19*(1), 41.

Women's International Network. (1994, Autumn). Egypt: UN conference on population and development and FGM. *Women's International Network News, 20*(4), 29.

Women's International Network. (1997, Autumn). Educational materials for prevention of FGM. Women's International Network News, 23(4), 23.

Women's International Network. (1998, Autumn). Action points: Follow-up to symposium on Addis Ababa for Legislators. *Women's International Network News, 24*(4), 29.

Women's International Network. (1999, Winter). Female Genital Mutilation . . . Is the ban effective in Ghana? *Women's International Network News, 25*(1), 32.

Printed in the United Kingdom by
Lightning Source UK Ltd., Milton Keynes
140199UK00001B/11/P